At the Heart of St. Mary's

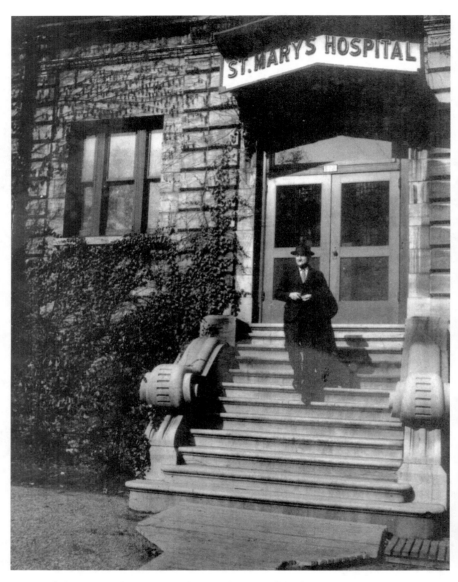

Radiologist Dr. John Cecil Lanthier on the steps of the first St. Mary's Hospital in Shaughnessey House, 1926.

At the Heart
of St. Mary's

A History of Montreal's
St. Mary's Hospital Center

ALAN HUSTAK

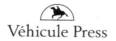

Véhicule Press

Published with the assistance of the Canada Council for the Arts, the
Canada Book Fund of the Department of Canadian Heritage, and the
Société de développement des entreprises culturelles du Québec (SODEC).

Cover design: David Drummond
Typeset in Minion by David LeBlanc
Printed by Marquis Printing Inc.

Library and Archives Canada Cataloguing in Publication
Hustak, Alan, 1944–, author
At the heart of St. Mary's : a history of Montreal's St. Mary's
Hospital Center / Alan Hustak.

Includes index.
ISBN 978-1-55065-361-8 (pbk.)
1. St. Mary's Hospital (Montréal, Québec)—History. 2. Hospitals—
Québec (Province)—Montréal—History. I. Title.
RA983.M6S36 2013   362.1109714'28   C2013-905910-5

Published by Véhicule Press, Montréal, Québec, Canada
www.vehiculepress.com

Distribution in Canada by LitDistCo
www.litdistco.ca

Distributed in the U.S. by Independent Publishers Group
www.ipgbook.com

Printed in Canada on FSC certified paper

A hospital must not only render the most efficient service to the sick; it must have a heart as well. It must realize that a patient is a human being, a creature in God's likeness, and as such, be accorded kindness and consideration.
St. Mary's is such a hospital.
~ Georges Gauthier, Archbishop of Montreal

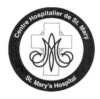

This book is dedicated to the patients at St. Mary's and to their
families, who for eight decades have trusted the hospital to deliver
quality and compassionate care; to the Irish community that built it,
to the nuns that ran it, to the support staff and volunteers who
continue to sustain its spirit, to the medical students and trainees
who serve to challenge and move the hospital forward, to its various
boards, and to all of those who, through their leadership
and commitment, continue to enrich St. Mary's
by their loyalty and their expertise.

CONTENTS

FOREWORD

ᔖ

This book is the direct result of an appeal from a number of members of the St. Mary's Hospital Center family who have such an attachment to the place that they were determined to see its extraordinary history preserved. Dr. J.J. Dinan wrote the first book, *St. Mary's Hospital: The Early Years*, in 1987.

From its stormy beginnings as a faith-based institution in the 1920s, through its expansion during the Depression, up until its official recognition by the Ministry as a university-affiliated hospital centre in this century, there has been a human dimension to St. Mary's that has not always been easy to achieve in an institutional setting.

The history of the hospital is, above all, one of extraordinary devotion – by those who built it, work for it, and support its unique role in the community. The story told here not only celebrates its medical achievements but also chronicles the rivalries and ongoing struggles that ensured its survival. At the same time, it recognizes the contributions of the doctors, nuns, nurses, other healthcare professionals, staff, and, of course, the countless volunteers who, from the hospital's very beginnings, have always been committed to excellence in healthcare.

St. Mary's has been a part of my life since I first arrived here in 1972 as a summer extern. I returned in 1974 as a rotating intern with $35 in my pocket. I was privileged not only to work at St. Mary's, but also to guide its fortunes for the last 16 years as its director general and chief executive officer. St. Mary's is not perfect, and while it is not always easy to be part of the public health system these days, I am especially proud that St. Mary's is consistently recognized as one of the most performant hospitals on the Island of Montreal.

On a personal note, it has been a pleasure and a privilege to be associated with the hospital throughout my professional career. On behalf of everyone at the hospital, I want to recognize the thousands of students from all health disciplines who have done part of their training at St. Mary's. We are a better place because of them. I want to particularly thank the generations of patients and families for placing their trust in St. Mary's and for the privilege of having been able to serve them.

I would be remiss if I did not recognize the four people who were passionate about this project: Doctors Guy Joron, Richard Moralejo, Constant Nucci, and James Sullivan. Of course, my special thanks to Alan Hustak for writing the book and Véhicule Press for publishing it.

As a new generation of administrators prepares to step into the future, I hope this history serves not only as a reminder of the hospital's past but also helps them, during times of inevitable change, to guard and preserve the indelible identity that is St. Mary's.

ARVIND K. JOSHI, M.D.
Montreal, Quebec

PREFACE

࢟

In January 1930, with the economy shrinking, Dr. Donald Hingston, the ambitious son of a knighted Montreal surgeon, set out to raise $1 million to build a hospital to serve Montreal's Irish Catholics. It was an audacious initiative, but gradually the Irish community supported Hingston's endeavours and, in spite of the Depression, people chipped in, brick by brick, to build a community hospital. In 1934, St. Mary's Hospital opened at its present location, 3830 Lacombe Avenue.

Hingston was a man of uncommon energy and ambition. It took a great deal of bargaining and resolve to keep the hospital operating, and, in spite of the constant strain this placed on him over the years, Hingston succeeded. Thanks to the generosity of volunteers, the largesse of benefactors, and government money, St. Mary's Hospital Center has not only survived, but, since its ministerial designation as a university-affiliated hospital centre in 2008, it has also become Montreal's leading community hospital.

Five years ago, during the twelfth official recession in 80 years, the hospital once again embarked on an audacious initiative: this time it would raise $120 million for an infrastructure renewal plan to face the challenges of the twenty-first century. The plans include the addition of two new floors on the West Wing, renovations and expansion of the critical care units, more operating suites on the second floor and the rebuilding of 5300 Côte-des-Neiges as a state-of-the-art office building for physicians' offices and clinics associated with the hospital. Unlike the multibillion dollar super-hospital projects – encompassing the

Centre hospitalier de l'Universite de Montréal (CHUM) and the McGill University Health Centre (MUHC) – which, at this writing, is enmeshed in administrative scandal and cost overruns – the St. Mary's project is quietly moving ahead in phases. "St. Mary's needs the space, it's that simple," says Ralph Dadoun, St. Mary's vice president of corporate and support services. "We have no control over the number of people who go through our emergency rooms. Patient care could degrade with time."

Ten years ago, such an expansion would have been unthinkable. But St. Mary's has a history of overcoming the improbable. "We have an institution started by an Irish Catholic community and a clique of Irish Catholic doctors that was then run, and run well, for 50 years by Roman Catholic nuns, then by Bill Busat, then by a doctor of Italian [Canadian] descent; and now an East Indian Hindu with an MBA, who was educated in Ireland, speaks eight languages and is married to a Quebecer, is running the place," explains former board chairman, Richard Renaud, the financier and creative philanthropist who has been instrumental in shaping the hospital's future. The rationale behind the expansion, according to Renaud, is part of the hospital's natural evolution. "It is about continuing to provide quality health-care, and to provide quality care today is a different kind of game than it once was. The brand recognition around hospitals is over," he insists. "There are no longer Roman Catholic hospitals, Protestant hospitals, Jewish hospitals or ethnic hospitals. There are only community hospitals. And the best way for St. Mary's to excel as a community hospital is to make a statement of excellence, to build on the specific strengths in which it excels. It is one of the largest birthing centres, with about 5,000 maternity cases a year. It specializes in cataract surgery, it provides the most humane primary and secondary cancer care, and it has the most efficient and effective laboratories in the province, by any benchmark. It is one of Quebec's best-run hospitals. Its expansion is all about good governance."

Writing about an institution like St. Mary's is a daunting task. Everyone who has ever worked or been a patient there has a story to tell about the hospital. Those who believe in the place believe in it devoutly. It serves an immediate population of 233,000 in the most densely populated and multicultural of twelve Centres de santé et des services sociaux (CSSS) in the Montreal area. This book is a popular account of St. Mary's Hospital Center from its dubious beginnings in 1924 to the present day. It is by no means an academic or a definitive history, since the hospital's archives have been sorely neglected and have never been properly catalogued. I am grateful that Dr. Jack Dinan wrote about the hospital 20 years before me. His slim but useful memoir, *St. Mary's Hospital: The Early Years*, was the foundation for this book. I was not totally unfamiliar with the hospital's beginnings, however, having touched on the story in my 2004 biography of Sir William Hingston.

Great institutions are forged by dynamic leaders, and I was fortunate to be able to interview a number of them for this book, including doctors David Kahn, Guy Joron, Richard Moralejo, and Constant Nucci, who enriched its pages with their insights, and Monsignor Sean Harty and Dr. Arvind K. Joshi, who were there when things took longer than expected. I thank them all for their patience. Similarly, Alain Benedetti and Richard Renaud shed light on some dark passages. Much of the material for this account comes from the minutes of the hospital's Board of Directors and from the annual reports, to which I was given unrestricted access.

The Sisters of Providence, the Grey Nuns, and the Hospitalières de Saint-Joseph were extremely forthcoming with pertinent material from their archives, as were Gilles Teasdale, Marjolaine Martel, and Anthony Mullins at the St. Mary's Hospital Center library and photo archives.

The unpublished diaries of doctors Donald Hingston and Emmett Mullally, who were there from the start, added texture. The Osler Library of the History of Medicine at McGill University and the *Canadian Medical Association Journal* proved to be invaluable. Special thanks to Nancy Marrelli, archivist emerita at the Concordia University archives and long-time member of the St. Mary's Hospital Board,

Gordon Burr at the McGill University archives, Louise Verdant at the Musée des Hospitalières de l'Hôtel-Dieu de Montréal, Mylène Laurendeau and Hélène Leblond, archivists with the Grey Nuns in Montreal, and Gayle Desarmia and Danielle Hughes, archivists with the Sisters of Providence of St. Vincent de Paul in Kingston, Ontario. To the many doctors who spoke with me, or family members who wrote to me, or otherwise offered help, my deepest appreciation. Among them were: Ralph Dadoun, John Keyserlingk, Ben Thompson, Peter Gruner, Mark J. Yaffe, Gerald Berry, Tom Altimas, Peter Duffy, Joe Dylewski, Peter McCracken, José Rodriguez, Mrs. Karl Essig, Jeffrey Kwitko, Daisy Pick, Richard Cruess, David Shaffelburg, Yosh Taguchi, Sandra Dolan, Peter Howlett, Andy Gutkowski, and, especially, Jim Sullivan, who nudged things along and who, with Dr. Guy Joron, offered advice over a number of pleasant dinners at Le Béarn. My only regret is that Guy didn't live to see the manuscript completed. He died in 2011.

Thanks also to Danielle Robitaille, Dan Burke, Caroline Emblem, Charlotte French, Nicole Tinmouth, Maureen Fitzgerald, Maureen Rappaport, Margaret O'Hanley, Brian Gallery, Jay Gould, Betty Ann Huberdeau, Edna Johns, Mrs. Janet Macklem, Helene McCormack, Patricia McDougall, Jane Skelton Mullally, Helen Lanthier, Patrick Wickham, Brian O'Neill, John Pepper, and Desmond Clarke, all of whom shared pertinent family papers or directed me to original source material of which I might otherwise have been unaware. My research was assisted by Lucinda Boyd in Chicago, Cynda P. Heward and Sheila Aronoff at the St. Mary's Hospital Foundation, Hugh Whalen, Barbara Bourne, Patricia Bennett, Lucile Lavigueur, Nick Beshwaty, Elizabeth Gibson, Mary Lynne Desbarats, Julie Plamondon, Jean Mahoney, Dominic Taddeo, Robert Vanden Abeele, Suzanne Brosseau, Stanley Drummond, Viviane Tawil, Patrick Letang; and Sonia Grégoire at the Lakeshore General Hospital. I also thank *Gazette* librarians Michael Porritt, Patricia Duggan, and David Pinto; Eric Durocher at the *Catholic Times*; and Beryl Wajsman, who not only gave me a hat but also a place to hang it.

I of course thank the St. Mary's Hospital Center and the Hospital Foundation for commissioning this book, and I am even more grateful that the hospital staff left me alone, without interference, to write it. Whatever the book's shortcomings, I alone am responsible for its content and its interpretation of the facts. Thanks to Mary Williams for editing the manuscript. Once again, it has been a great pleasure to work with Simon Dardick and his team at Véhicule Press. I value his expertise, judgement, candour, advice, and especially his friendship.

Montreal – Montebello
July 2013
AMDG

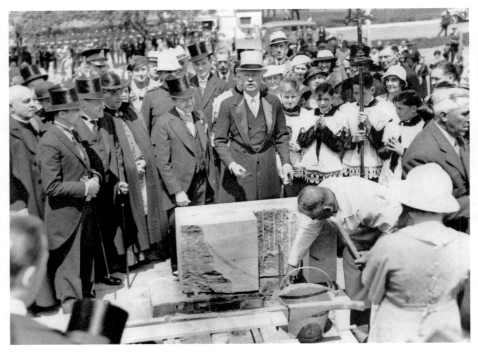

Governor General Bessborough (centre) places the cornerstone for St. Mary's Hospital, June 17, 1933, as Thomas Taggart Smyth, president of the hospital's Board of Directors, looks on.

INTRODUCTION

Doctors, politicians in their silk top hats, parish priests, curates in ecclesiastical robes, nuns in their itchy black habits, and an unusual number of women gathered in an open field at the corner of Lacombe Avenue and Côte-des-Neiges Road in Montreal on Saturday, June 17, 1933. In spite of the threat of rain, this crowd had assembled during the cruellest year of the Depression to witness the laying of the cornerstone of St. Mary's Memorial Hospital, a facility designed to serve Montreal's English-speaking population. Among those who had made their way to the site were Mayor Fernand Rinfret, who had been secretary of state in Prime Minister Mackenzie King's Cabinet, Joseph Henry Dillon, member of the Quebec legislature for the largely Irish constituency of St. Ann's, and Thomas Taggart Smyth, public-spirited general manager of the Montreal City and District Savings Bank and president of the hospital's Board of Directors. Cadets from Collège Mont-St-Louis provided the royal salute as Canada's 14th governor general, British aristocrat Vere Brabazon Ponsonby, the 9th Earl of Bessborough, arrived to place the stone. Cached inside the cornerstone were coins, memorabilia, and newspapers of the day – which, among other things, were reporting that the United States dollar had reached "its lowest level in memory," President Franklin Delano Roosevelt was vacationing at his mother's home in Campobello, New Brunswick, Canada's prime minister, Richard Bedford Bennett, was on his way to an economic summit in England, and Quebec's Liberal premier,

Louis-Alexandre Taschereau, was promising to help the vast numbers of those without jobs "by means of public works instead of direct relief."

Everywhere there were signs of disease and malnutrition, breadlines and unemployment. Bessborough dedicated the building "to those who seek relief from suffering" and asked that "the blessing of God rest upon those who will work within its walls." But Montreal's portly Roman Catholic bishop, Georges Gauthier, who offered the blessing, didn't seem worried about hard times. "I am not much concerned about the present economic crisis or its effect on our population," the Bishop declared. "I don't need to remind you that Montreal is, geographically speaking, a pretty big city with a reputation of being among the foremost cities in commerce and industry. But it occupies no less an honourable position in the world of charity. I deeply rejoice that another charitable institution is about to take its place among the many institutions like it that we enjoy." The *Gazette* reported that while the new medical facility would be "owned and operated by English-speaking Catholics, it will be a general hospital open to all citizens regardless of race, creed or circumstance."

Getting the hospital built had not been easy. An institution for English-speaking Roman Catholics hadn't been much of a priority for the overwhelmingly French-speaking diocese. Initial attempts in 1924 to open a temporary hospital without essential government support had proven to be an embarrassment. Those directly involved sparred over the creation of St. Mary's, and often the prospect of getting it off the ground seemed impossible. Dr. Donald Hingston, the hospital's surgeon-in-chief, who was lost in the crowd that day, promoted the idea and secured the necessary financial support from the city and the province. The stock market crash of 1929 forced those concerned to amend the plans, but the hospital was built. Certainly, those responsible for St. Mary's Memorial Hospital had high ideals. An early operational handbook spelled out that while it was to be a Roman Catholic institution, it was in every way designed as a community hospital, "open to all, rich or poor, irrespective of race, creed or financial condition." All patients were to be treated equally, regardless of status or income. The hospital's code of ethics was later enunciated by Hingston: "The ideal of friendship and fairness among the members of the staff; the ideal of unfailing courtesy and respect towards the nursing sisters and patients, the ambition that the members of the staff will be looked up to scientifically and professionally, and that financial success will always be held secondary to professional success."

The original plans for the hospital had been drawn up in 1932 by Henry Walsh, a Chicago consultant, and they were patterned after those of the Passavant Memorial Hospital, which had opened to the carriage trade in June 1929. Passavant was located in one of Chicago's most affluent neighbourhoods, the Near North Side, and it was intended to serve that neighbourhood. Extensive wood panelling, subdued lighting, and comfortable chairs in the waiting area created an atmosphere of dignified quiet. Walsh's elaborate Gothic-Jacobean design for St. Mary's – a seven-storey building with two towers, one housing a domed chapel and the other a solarium with a panoramic view of the city – proved to be too palatial. During the Depression, the design was scaled down by a Montreal architect, Edward J. Turcotte, who was also responsible for a number of hospital buildings in Brome-Missisquoi, Quebec, and in the Maritimes. Turcotte, incidentally, is the same architect responsible for the Church of the Ascension in Westmount.

If St. Mary's resembled a first-class railway hotel when it opened, it is perhaps because John Archibald, who worked on the project for two years before his death in 1934, had designed a number of hotels for the Canadian National Railway. Its main entrance was on Lacombe Avenue. Two marble staircases led to the main lobby on the first floor, with its graceful Jacobean-period mezzanine and decorative coffered ceiling. The first floor housed the executive and administrative offices, a chapel, rooms for eight interns, the hospital's laboratories – cardiography, pathology, and bacteriology – and the hospital's main kitchen.

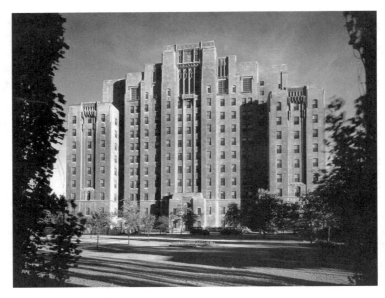

Chicago's Passavant Memorial Hospital opened in 1929.

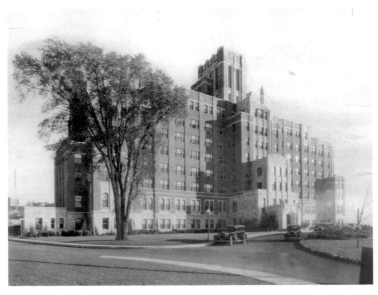

Montreal's St. Mary's Hospital Center opened in 1934.

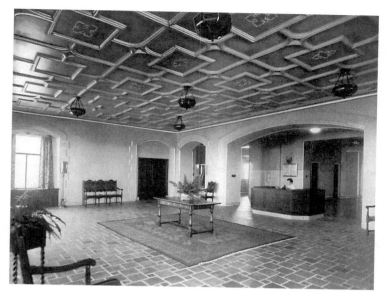

The original main lobby, 1934.

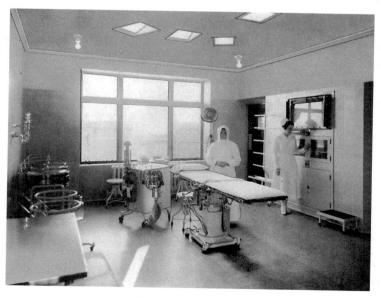

State-of-the-art operating theatre, 1934.

On the ground floor, there was also an outpatient department, an emergency unit, and an operating room, which Turcotte described as unique, in that patients are brought in through a covered ambulance entrance, a feature not usually found in the average hospital.

On the second floor were the public wards, the largest with six beds, but most of them with four – this at a time when all the other hospitals in the city offered public wards of 12 to 36 beds. Brightly lit private deluxe suites were on the third floor, each decorated in a pearl-grey-and-green colour scheme and containing colour-coordinated furniture, which made them "cheerful and home-like." Each floor had its own service kitchen, nursing station, solarium, flower room, and linen room. Five state-of-the-art operating theatres with terrazzo floors and scrub rooms were situated on the fourth floor – three for general surgery, one with a Holly table for orthopedics, and one for genitourinary procedures. The lights in the operating theatre "cast absolutely no shadow and threw no heat; these are very important points, and the latest developments in operating room lighting." The recovery rooms were also on the fourth floor.

The entire fifth floor was the Maternity Wing, with 30 beds and 30 bassinets, and "every facility for the convenience of patients." Thirty nurses lived on the sixth floor. A pediatric department accommodating 30 children occupied the West Wing of the seventh floor, and the cloisters for the nursing sisters were in the East Wing. Two enclosed rooftop solariums were also on the eighth floor, and two open terraces with panoramic views of a large corner of Lake St-Louis and Lake of Two Mountains to the west, St. Joseph's Oratory (still under construction) to the south, and to the east, the Laurentian Mountains and beyond to the rooftops of St-Jérôme. All corridors and public rooms were soundproofed, making the hospital exceptionally quiet. Only the soothing sound of xylophones, which were played at each nursing station to summon the interns, broke the stillness. As one intern recalled, "They gave certain signals: in C-major for residents and E-minor for junior interns. National anthems and pop tunes were excluded from intonation but bars of hymns allowed."

The hospital's electrical equipment, turbo generators, and a self-contained emergency battery-operated supply system were housed behind the hospital in a separate building designed to resemble a tower. As the architect Turcotte boasted, "Each floor is a complete hospital in itself, which means that St. Mary's really comprises several hospitals under one roof, one of the most modern and best-equipped hospitals of its size on the continent."

The hospital had its own 24-hour ambulance and emergency service, and all doctors with privileges could admit their private patients to St. Mary's. While the hospital was still under construction, 12 medical departments were established and staff doctors appointed. The largest of these were Obstetrics and Gynecology, Pediatrics, Medicine, and Surgery. Others included Anesthesia, Neurology, Dermatology, Ophthalmology, Pathology, Nose and Throat, Dentistry, and Roentgenology (X-ray department). St. Mary's, also designed to operate an outpatient clinic and a social services department, was certified by the American College of Surgeons as a grade A general hospital.

Premier Taschereau and Montreal's mayor, Camillien Houde, were among the dignitaries who attended the formal dedication of St. Mary's on Sunday, November 24, 1934. "If the poor are always with us, the sick are their inheritance," hospital board president Taggart Smyth told the assembled guests. With that, Bishop Gauthier, who was 600 kilometres away in Woonsocket, Rhode Island, pressed a button, and at precisely 3:12 p.m., the main doors electronically swung open. Smyth then enunciated what has since become the hospital's mission statement: "The door of St. Mary's has no lock. Now that our doors are open they can never close. They will remain open twenty-four hours a day to the sick and injured of all races, all creeds and all colours."

To those who believe in such things, the miracle was that the doors had opened at all.

CHAPTER ONE

St. Mary's. It is the wonderful name of our Lord's blessed mother and
is sufficiently universal ever to be parochial. I like the name.
~ Thomas Taggart Smyth

ॐ

St. Mary's exists because of two people: a well-heeled young surgeon
and a belligerent nun. When others said there weren't enough English-
speaking Catholics in Montreal to support a hospital of their own,
Donald Hingston and Helen Morrissey drove the project forward with
little more than their sheer determination.

Morrissey, a nursing sister, met Hingston in 1901 when they worked
together at Hôtel-Dieu de Montréal, the city's oldest hospital for
French-speaking patients. Founded by Jeanne Mance in 1644, the
hospital had been run efficiently for almost two and a half centuries
by a religious nursing order, the Hospitalières de St-Joseph. The sisters were well experienced in directing hospitals, and they understood
the enormous potential of linking cures for the body with a faith that
offered a cure for the soul.

Helen Morrissey was born into a Roman Catholic family in Pick-
ering, Ontario, on May 28, 1860. She was educated at Protestant
schools and at the Ontario Ladies' College. Much to her parents' dis-
may, in 1885, she joined the Hospitalières to become a nursing sister.
She was a zealous romantic, and, according to her fellow sisters,
"someone with lofty aims and Napoleonic ambition." Morrissey's
biographer, Jeanne Lama, describes her as "saintly, womanly, coura-
geous, yet often impractical." It is perhaps telling that Morrissey took
as one of her role models Frances Margaret "Fanny" Allen, the rebel-
lious daughter of the storied American Revolutionary War hero, Ethan
Allen. Fanny's father established Vermont's Green Mountain Boys,

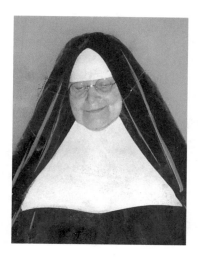

Sister Helen Morrissey, first
Superior of St. Mary's.

invaded Quebec in 1775, and was captured by the British. Against his
wishes, his daughter rejected a marriage proposal and became a nun.
She entered the Hospitalières order in 1808 and spent 11 years in a
cloistered sisterhood as the hospital's chemist before her death in 1819.
Helen Morrissey, too, directed the hospital's pharmacy. As one of only
two English-speaking nuns at Hôtel-Dieu, she had easy access to the
leaders of Montreal's English-speaking community. Her talent was as
a fundraiser. She built "a network of generous benefactors" and trans-
formed Hôtel-Dieu's outdated dispensary into a department that was
"the object of admiration by authorities of other hospitals."

When Morrissey started working at Hôtel-Dieu, it had only two
telephones: one in the entry hall, the other in the cloister. Not only did
she persuade Bell to give the hospital its first 30 telephones, but she
also got the company to waive the hospital's annual $750 telephone
bill. Similarly, she organized a fundraising drive that yielded $10,000 –
more than enough to buy "two of the most beautiful carriages and
four of the most beautiful horses in the city" for the hospital's first
ambulance service.

Donald Hingston arrived at Hôtel-Dieu in 1901 as a 23-year-old
intern after graduating in medicine from Université Laval à Montréal.

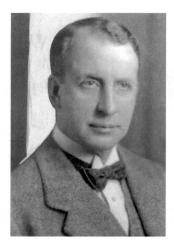

Donald Hingston, founder of St. Mary's.

He came to work with his father, Sir William Hingston, the hospital's chief surgeon, who had been mayor of Montreal in the 1870s, and who had been knighted in 1895 by Queen Victoria for his contributions to modern surgery before being appointed to the Canadian Senate. His son, Donald, was a young man of tremendous drive and ambition. At Hôtel-Dieu, the younger Hingston became increasingly concerned about the way in which the needs of English-speaking patients were being ignored. He spent his residency in England where, in 1903, he was admitted to the Royal College of Surgeons. In his absence, Sister Morrissey had taken it upon herself to renovate St. Bridget's ward, which housed Hôtel-Dieu's English-speaking female patients. She was knowledgeable about antique furniture. While redecorating, she found a valuable 17th-century Louis XIII-style table that had been covered with so many coats of paint that it was unrecognizable. She had it restored, and it can still be found in the common room of the Hospitalières' motherhouse. By the time she had finished redecorating, the ward was so luxurious that people had begun referring to it as "the White House."

English Catholics in Montreal had been without a hospital of their own for nearly 50 years, ever since the small, short-lived St. Patrick's

Hospital had shut its doors. St. Patrick's was opened in 1852, but it was absorbed by the Hospitalières – occupying two wards of their vast new Hôtel-Dieu building – in 1860, when the order consolidated all of its facilities on Pine Avenue. Once that happened, almost 40 percent of Montreal's English Catholics had to depend on the city's three Protestant hospitals: the Royal Victoria Hospital, which opened on the slopes of Mount Royal in 1894; Western Hospital, a privately funded institution, which opened in 1876; and the Montreal General Hospital, which traces its beginnings to 1821.

These Protestant hospitals were not receptive to having Catholic interns or nurses on staff, and McGill University wasn't especially welcoming to Roman Catholics on campus. "Catholic students at McGill, although living in a Catholic city, were left to themselves as far as the practice of their religion," wrote Emmett Mullally, who had come from Souris West, Prince Edward Island, in 1897 to study medicine at McGill. "There was always the danger of our faith becoming lukewarm through the insidious attacks which half-baked professors made upon the religion." To complete their medical training, young English-speaking Roman Catholic graduates like Mullally often had to leave Quebec. Those who could afford to went to Europe.

Although Protestant hospitals admitted Roman Catholics as interns and patients, they discouraged Catholics from practising their religion on the premises, making it difficult for priests to hear confession, deliver communion, or administer the last sacraments to the dying. French-speaking Catholics in Montreal had two hospitals. In addition to Hôtel-Dieu, there was Hôpital Notre-Dame, which had been set up in 1880 by Université Laval. A hospital for English-speaking Catholics in the city was long overdue.

Initially, Hingston and Morrissey got along well. Hingston liked Morrissey's strong personality and especially admired her talent as "an exceptionally fine collector of money." Both believed that no matter how good the facilities at Hôtel-Dieu, the psychological well-being of its English-speaking patients was compromised within an institution that operated exclusively in French. These patients, as Morrissey put it, "could not die in English." She agreed with Hingston that the money she had spent on renovations could have been put to better use creating a new hospital. Very few records of the process that initiated the St. Mary's project exist, so it is hard to know just whose idea it really was. One thing is clear: the combined connections and impassioned drive of Hingston and Morrissey cannot be ignored. Undeniably, it was Morrissey who, with the approval of her superior, pushed ahead and started knocking on doors and collecting money. The Hospitalières were a fluid force in the city. They had the power to establish a new footing for their order wherever it was needed, which is precisely what Morrissey intended. In fact, in French-language histories, it is the Hospitalières who are credited as the founders of St. Mary's. Hingston dreamed of a hospital; Morrissey envisioned building a nursing school of her own to staff it.

The proposal remained in limbo for several years, until 1907, when Sir William Hingston died. Donald Hingston became a director of the Montreal City and District Savings Bank, of which Sir William had been president. The first tentative steps toward building a hospital were taken in the autumn of 1908, when Hingston invited a small group of movers and shakers to dinner. Not only had he lost his father, but he had also lost his younger sister, Aileen, who had died the previous year. To honour their memory, he proposed building the Sir William Hingston Memorial Hospital. From day one, Hingston envisioned a hospital run with a particular catholic hospitality, in the universal sense of the word. Above all, it would be a private institution "whose outstanding feature is gentle catholic charity in its truest sense," directed by a secular board that was out of reach of the institutional church, but would represent the Roman Catholic Church "absolutely and without hesitation." Hingston had good reason to distrust the institutional church. Sir William, a number of his father's fellow doctors at Hôtel-Dieu's School of Medicine and Surgery, and some of the students at the school had been excommunicated in 1883 for refusing to sever their ties with Victoria College, a Protestant university in Ontario, and accept instead positions at a satellite campus of Université Laval, a Roman Catholic institution that Archbishop Édouard-Charles Fabre was then trying to get off the ground in Montreal. The excommunication was suspended only after the doctors appealed to the Pope. The biggest obstacle to the dream of a hospital for English-speaking Catholics, however, was Archbishop Fabre's successor, the formidable Louis-Joseph-Napoléon-Paul Bruchési.

At the beginning of the twentieth century, the Roman Catholic Church in Quebec was a state within a state. It functioned as a social service as well as a religious institution and diocese; it administered and directed every aspect of the cultural, educational, medical, and social welfare of its parishioners. Without Bruchési's support, the entire project would have come to nothing. Coincidentally, Bruchési was at the time preoccupied with building Hôpital Notre-Dame on Sherbrooke Street, an institution for French-speaking patients. English-speaking parishioners numbered about 15,000 in a city of 200,000 French-speaking residents. To Bruchési, the needs of so small a minority were not a priority. Hingston explored alternative avenues. He sought help from the Sulpicians, the original *seigneurs* of the Island of Montreal, who still held sway, but they turned him down. In 1913, Hingston travelled to Toronto to see whether the Sisters of the Order of St. Joseph would be interested in helping him. "They asked me point-blank whether Bruchési would welcome them. I told them that if they wanted an honest answer, they would not be welcome, but we could take up the matter strongly with the papal delegate." The sisters considered the request and decided they weren't interested. An economic downturn and widespread financial uncertainty further stalled plans for a hospital, and the idea was shelved indefinitely when the First World War began in 1914. Hingston enlisted in the medical corps and went overseas with the Irish Rangers. While he was away, Sister Morrissey opened St. Ann's Dispensary, a small medical clinic on Eleanor Street in Griffintown. It handled about 6,000 patients a year, but it was hardly what either of them had imagined as a hospital.

In the autumn of 1916, Hingston returned from Europe to teach embryology at Université Laval à Montreal. "His methods of teaching were different from those of his colleagues," one of his students recalled. "As an anatomist, he knew topography and histology thoroughly. His memory never failed him. He conducted his clinics by the question-and-answer method. Time was of no consequence. When called in consultation, Dr. Hingston remained calm and never rendered a hasty decision. In his opinion, it was always better to adhere to the well-known practice of 'wait and see' rather than give a doubtful decision." He was fond of quoting Voltaire's maxim: "The art of medicine consists of amusing the patient while nature cures the disease."

The symbolic beginning of St. Mary's was October 10, 1916, when Hingston convened a meeting at the University Club to revive the idea of building a hospital. Among those present that night were a former provincial Cabinet minister, Dr. James John Guerin, who had been the mayor of Montreal from 1910 to 1912. Hingston regarded Guerin as "a noisy show-off, but an important ally." Another original supporter was Dr. Francis Devlin, medical superintendent of Hôpital St-Jean-de-Dieu (a psychiatric hospital) and the city's leading psychiatrist, or "alienist," as they were called in those days. In Hingston's eyes, Devlin was "a whole-hearted fighter, a man of charming personality, artistic, very musical, an outstanding debater with rapier-like repartee, and an idealist thoroughly loyal to his ideals, a true sincere Catholic, an honourable man who possessed a very clear vision." Then there was Dr. John Leo Delany Mason, who graduated from McGill in 1903, served as a captain in the Royal Canadian Army Medical Corps during the First World War, and then returned to McGill to teach pharmacology. Like Devlin, Mason was an eloquent and persuasive speaker and pledged to do all he could to promote the hospital. Also present was Dr. Joseph James "Mac" McGovern from Danville, Quebec, who taught school by day, studied dermatology by night, and opened his own private practice in Pointe-St-Charles – an inner-city neighbourhood where most of the Irish poor lived – after graduating from Bishop's University's medical school in 1904. "That night the torch was lighted, there was an enthusiasm and a fine feeling of determination to succeed against all opposition," Hingston recorded in his diary.

Helen Morrissey wasn't at the meeting. But, at Hingston's suggestion, and "remembering the long debt of gratitude the English-speaking Catholics owe the sisters of the Hôtel-Dieu," it was resolved that Morrissey be put in charge of internal management and nursing at the proposed new hospital. The hospital itself would, they decreed, be "directed and maintained" by a secular board of governors. "We make this request…with full confidence of a very successful future," the board informed Morrissey's superior, Sister Ste-Thérèse, on November 1. "If your community will join us in this undertaking, we can promise you a full and loyal support and cooperation."

On November 16, Archbishop Bruchési consented to the arrangement on the condition that the diocese would not be involved. He gave his blessing to those sisters "who so desire to devote themselves to this good work and to form their own autonomous community with nursing sisters from other orders who have permission from their superiors to join them. If, after having considered all aspects of the question, your order agrees in principle to accept the offer, I have no objection. You are free to decide for yourselves." Bruchési made it clear, however, that final permission would have to come from Rome.

Bruchési was not keen on the idea of appointing Morrissey as head of the nursing school. "She is not the person you want," he warned Hingston. "She is not practical. She means well, but she lacks the fundamental Christian virtue of charity." Morrissey lived in a cloistered world of Latin song and prayer, incense and sacraments, and had little or no experience in business administration. She reviewed the doctors' offer, and, wary of finding herself in a position where she would be subservient to a secular board, informed the doctors that she refused to place the "religious life, rules, and regulations the sisters must follow" under lay control. Nursing sisters under her supervision, she argued, must be compelled to obey the rules of the religious community she wished to start. Negotiations continued, and on December 29, after a meeting with Archbishop Bruchési, Hingston and Sister Ste-Thérèse agreed that "the expenses of the [religious] community" would be paid from "the Hospitalières' funds." In the event of a dispute between the sisters and the board, "the Bishop of Montreal would have the final word."

On January 19, 1917, the Hospitalières accepted the conditions and agreed to let its English-speaking sisters devote themselves to the work at hand. A rich widow, Mrs. James Cochrane, donated a handsome 10-room brownstone at 34 Hutchison Street, just above Sherbrooke Street, to serve as a hospital building. The house was worth $22,000. Because it was too small to be converted into a hospital, Morrissey sold it. She was ready to launch a major public fundraising campaign, but Bruchési suggested that the time for this was "inopportune" – she should wait until the war was over.

In 1918, Donald Hingston was appointed professor of embryology at Université de Montréal's Faculty of Medicine. He no longer had as much time to devote to the hospital project as he would have liked. The war ended that autumn, then an influenza epidemic closed schools and churches in the city. Other complications arose. Hingston's older brother, William, a Jesuit priest, had been named rector of Loyola College in the Montreal neighbourhood of Notre-Dame-de-Grâce. The school, which had opened in 1916, was bankrupt. William Hingston asked his brother to delay fundraising for the hospital until his own drive to raise $300,000 for Loyola was over. "A college of the type of Loyola is a necessity, it is evident the Catholic public cannot get on without it," William insisted. "The college comes first, a hospital will follow, and other works will come as a matter of course."

In mid-January, the doctors involved in the hospital project voted to postpone their fundraising efforts until Loyola had reached its objective. Taggart Smyth of the Montreal City and District Savings Bank joined the group later that spring. In May, a fundraising campaign for Loyola was launched, but the response to the appeal was disappointing. Setbacks continued. In 1919, Archbishop Bruchési lost his grip on reality, and the administration of the diocese was handed over to his auxiliary, Georges Gauthier. It would be necessary to repeat the whole process: Gauthier would have to be made familiar with the project, and his support for it would have to be won.

In a bid to secure financing, the board approached the most powerful lay Catholic in Canada: Lord Shaughnessy, the tightfisted, temperamental, American-born president of the Canadian Pacific Railway. Shaughnessy had been made a baron in 1916 for his services to king and country during the war. He was known for his incessant nit-picking, and the board members found their meeting with him quite memorable. "Shaughnessy mercilessly attacked all aspects of the project," wrote Hingston. "Was the hospital necessary? Have we the men? Could we get the money? Why have a religious hospital? He addressed the questions principally to me, and I answered as well as I could. His attack was almost bitter. Then, satisfied with our answers, his whole tone changed as he said, 'Gentlemen, I am with you.'"

Lord Shaughnessy agreed to become founding president of St. Mary's Hospital. He pledged $20,000 to the cause on the condition that all of the hospital directors be English-speaking Catholics. With Shaughnessy's support, St. Mary's obtained its corporate charter from the Quebec legislature on February 14, 1920. The charter was unusual for the time, in that it put management in the hands of a secular board of directors instead of the Church. The dual nature of the institution was spelled out in article 2 of Bill 82, the enabling legislation: St. Mary's would be a general hospital under Catholic control that would treat "sick and injured persons of all races and creeds without distinction," and at the same time give "instruction in nursing and grant certificates of competency to nurses."

The news should have been cause for jubilation, but circumstances surrounding the passing of the legislation caused a clash of egos that resulted in what was to be the first of many unpleasant episodes in the history of the hospital's management.

The legislature was scheduled to prorogue the same day Bill 82 was passed, but before it could become law, the government needed the names of the hospital's petitioners. Hingston was telephoned, and, off the top of his head, he supplied the names of Lord Shaughnessy; Judge Charles Doherty, the federal minister of justice; Frank Devlin, the Conservative member of Parliament for Montreal's Irish constituency,

St. Ann's; and Taggart Smyth. When the names were published the following morning, Dr. Guerin was apoplectic. Guerin had just announced that he would be running against Judge Doherty in the forthcoming federal election. Naming Doherty as a director, Guerin argued, would give Doherty an unfair political advantage. Hingston added Guerin's name to the list. No sooner had the revised list of petitioners been printed to include Guerin than Sister Morrissey arrived at Hingston's door "in a fury, in one of her most angry, unreasoning moods." She demanded to know why Guerin's name had been added and insisted that if his name was to be associated with the hospital, she no longer wanted any part of it. "She was adamant: Dr. Guerin's name was to be deleted or she would withdraw at once." Convinced that she had been deliberately snubbed, Morrissey convened a meeting of her superiors on May 9, 1920. With their backing, she strengthened her own leverage to force the board to do her bidding.

The hospital's first board of directors was named on November 15, 1920. Guerin was on it. In addition to Hingston, Devlin, and Smith, the board included Leo George Ryan, the founder of Monsanto Canada, who had made a fortune pioneering agricultural chemicals; William J. Daly, founding president of the manufacturing firm Daly and Morin; and Reverend Thomas O'Reilly, a soft-spoken diocesan priest who had been chaplain at Hôtel-Dieu off and on for 27 years. Rounding off the board was Judge Doherty. It didn't take long for even more serious conflicts to emerge among the various personalities involved.

The first order of business was financial: Sister Morrissey was asked to account for the money she had raised to build the hospital. Morrissey was evasive. She was not prepared to open her books until Rome had approved her nursing order. She assured the board that she had $150,000 for her nursing school but was not about to hand any of it over until the board itself had raised funds for the hospital. Furthermore, as long as her nemesis, Dr. Guerin, was on the board, she saw no reason to cooperate. Hingston turned to Father O'Reilly to see if the priest could reason with Morrissey. O'Reilly had a reputation as a "patient listener and a silent talker," but he, too, found dealing with Morrissey difficult. Hingston concluded, "the only thing to do was to expose the matter quite openly to Doctor Guerin, and ask him to withdraw." Guerin was "painfully hurt" by the suggestion and refused to quit. In the end, the board members voted 13 to 4 to satisfy Morrissey. They dismissed Guerin. "That most regrettable affair did us great harm," Hingston noted. "Guerin never forgave us and took no further part in helping the movement, but after that he never lost a chance to hurt us."

The contract between the Hospitalières, Sister Morrissey, and the St. Mary's Board of Directors, signed on May 10, 1921, was essentially the same agreement that had been hammered out with Bruchési five years earlier. It authorized Morrissey to establish her own religious community that would "co-operate in the running and administration of the hospital."

The final hurdle was removed on January 19, 1923, when Cardinal Camillo Laurenti, Prefect of the Sacred Congregation of Religious Orders in Rome, sanctioned the removal of the cloister from the new community of nursing sisters and put Sister Morrissey in charge as Reverend Mother Superior. Under the Vatican charter, Morrissey was entrusted not only to "give medical advice and medicines to the poor," but also to "give instruction and grant certificates of competency to nurses." A contract between Sister Morrissey and St. Mary's that was approved in February 1924 put Morrissey in charge of her own religious community and made it clear that if "a difference of opinion between the Board of Directors and Sister Morrissey should arise, the matter would be submitted to the Archbishop of Montreal, whose word would be final and binding on all parties."

Now head of her own religious community, Sister Morrissey seemed more manic than usual. That summer, she toured "the finest and best equipped" hospitals in Kingston, Toronto, Windsor, Detroit, Chicago, Minneapolis, Niagara, Hamilton, Cornwall, and Brockville. The report on her fact-finding mission filed on September 22 recommended that St. Mary's be patterned after either the Mayo Clinic

College of Medicine in Rochester, Minnesota, the Ford Hospital in Detroit, or St. Vincent Hospital in Chicago. All had floor plans that "were easy to supervise with fewer employees." She wanted St. Mary's to be "a light-tan or deep-red brick building, topped with a roof garden and sun balconies." Alarmed by her grandiose plans, the board passed another resolution, on November 29, 1923, demanding to know exactly how much money she had at her disposal. Again, Morrissey refused to open her books and said that she would guard her finances until the board decided where the hospital would be built. With that, events took another unexpected turn. Gerald McShane, the strong-willed and well-connected pastor of St. Patrick's Parish, joined the board and offered the directors $1 million and a large undeveloped tract of land near St. Patrick's Orphanage in Outremont, between Côte Ste Catherine Road and Wilderton Avenue, as a site for the hospital. There were, however, strings attached. McShane wanted Morrissey fired, and he wanted to have St. Patrick's Parish (which meant McShane himself) placed in charge of the proposed hospital. "Sister Morrissey's modest foundation, whatever its merits, is not compatible with the notion of a great hospital," he argued. "Her new community, with all its personnel, novices [and so on]…has taken upon itself a financial responsibility far beyond its means." McShane was prepared to reimburse the Hospitalières for money they had already invested to get St. Mary's off the ground, but on this point he was adamant: Morrissey must go.

It was a defining moment. Hingston was not about to surrender the board's autonomy to McShane, to the parish, or to the diocese. Whatever grief Morrissey had caused, Hingston had promised her that she would run the nursing school, and his word was his bond. McShane pointed out that the Vatican had changed regulations governing nuns working as nurses, and again he insisted that Morrissey be fired. The board voted in his favour. Hingston then threatened to resign if McShane's motion was allowed to stand. Again the board voted. This time, it reversed its earlier decision to oust Morrissey. It also reversed the previous motion to inspect Morrissey's books. Consequently, there

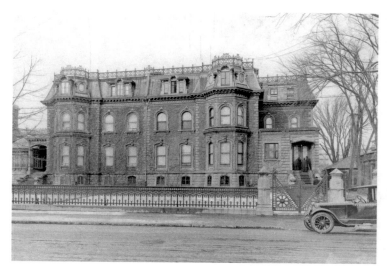

Shaughnessy House on Dorchester Boulevard, 1924 – the first
St. Mary's Hospital.

was now no way a financial statement could be tabled. Hingston
wrote: "The corporation [has] no funds on which to report, all dis-
bursements so far having been met by your directors personally."

Now fully in command, Morrissey took the directors by complete
surprise the following week when, acting on her own, she made a
$10,000 down payment on "temporary quarters at 1905 Dorchester
Street West in the residence of the late chairman, Lord Shaughnessy,"
who had died the previous year. With that, five of the directors, including McShane and Doherty, resigned in protest. When the *Gazette*
reported news of the resignations, Doherty denied that "there had
been anything in the way of trouble," and he urged the media not "to
create an impression that might hinder the good works which [could]
… be accomplished by the institution."

The 30-room mansion that Morrissey bought is today part of the
Canadian Centre for Architecture. Designed in the Second Empire
style by Montreal architect William Tutin Thomas, it had been built

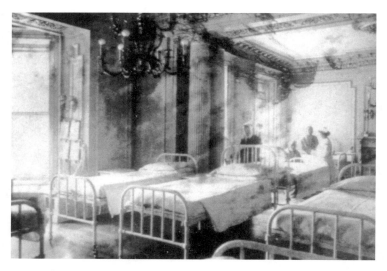

Chandeliers and opulence alone did not make a hospital ward.

as a sumptuous residence. Sir William Van Horne had lived in it in the 1880s when he was general manager of the Canadian Pacific Railway. After Shaughnessy moved in, in the 1890s, he commissioned architect Edward Maxwell to enlarge the premises. Hingston was not impressed with the building. He considered it "unsuitable for remodelling into a hospital." In spite of his misgivings, and without board approval, Morrissey took out a $55,000 mortgage on the mansion. Because women in Quebec at that time were not allowed to own property outright, the house was put in Father Thomas O'Reilly's name. With the deal a *fait accompli*, the board had little choice but to respect the contract it had signed with Morrissey. On May 15, 1923, she took possession. The following morning, Mass was celebrated in the dining room. "The splendour of the rich surroundings, tapestry, fixtures, carpets all added to the solemnity of the occasion," Morrissey wrote in her memoirs. "What a feeling of joy and thanksgiving was ours to think that Our Lord was now our first guest, and would remain with us to be our strength and support in trials."

According to the board minutes, Helen Morrissey was officially named as "first Superior and foundress of St. Mary's." Now Mother Morrissey, she was effectively the superior of a community with two other religious nurses, Bridget McCowan and Florence Campion. The next day, May 16, at the instigation of Mrs. James Cochrane, the St. Mary's Ladies Auxiliary was established at a founding meeting at the Windsor Hotel. Their mission was to help equip the hospital. Lady Margaret Hingston was elected first Auxiliary president. The formidable, 81-year-old Lady Hingston was a pious Catholic who wanted membership to be open to women from every parish and not restricted to women of means. In her acceptance speech, she railed against the parochial rivalries that threatened to undermine the success of the hospital. "Whereas sympathy is needed, co-operation is absolutely necessary," she said, insisting the executive include a representative "from each of the 16 English-speaking Roman Catholic parishes on the Island."

Aloysius Chopin became the hospital's first superintendent. There was no government funding for healthcare at the time, and he barely had "enough authority, assistance or enough money," to operate the hospital properly. Chopin, born in India of British parents, had fought with the British Army during the First World War. He was brought to Canada in 1919 to act as tutor for the children of industrialist Wilfrid Laurier McDougald, a medical doctor, who was then president of the Montreal Harbour Commission. (McDougald was also largely credited with getting the federal government to build the Jacques Cartier Bridge across the St. Lawrence River.)

For the most part, hospitals at that time depended on patients to pay their own medical costs; however, under the Quebec Public Charities Act, they were given $1.10 a day for each welfare patient they treated – about one-third of what the treatment cost. Only four of the rooms at St. Mary's were private. If the hospital were to continue, volunteers would be an essential cornerstone. Shortfalls in the operating budget would have to be made up by public subscription and fundraising campaigns.

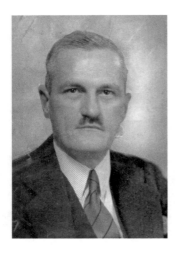

Dr. Wesley Bourne, St. Mary's
first anesthesiologist.

Five attending staff doctors administered the medical organization
of the hospital. Hingston was the surgeon-in-chief. Others on the first
medical board were Leo Mason, an attendee of the original 1908
founding meeting who had recently returned from doing postgraduate work in Paris; Emmett Mullally, "the man from the Island," an
amateur historian who had graduated from McGill in 1901 and who
had served with Hingston in the First World War as a medical officer
with the Irish Rangers; Jack C. Wickham, an abdominal surgery specialist; and Henry Robert Dunstan Gray, an obstetrician who ran his
own maternity clinic, Gray's Private Hospital. Thomas J. Gaslin, a
compact, compassionate 24-year-old intern from Green Valley,
Ontario, fresh from the University of Toronto, was engaged to handle admissions. Gaslin was required to be on duty for 16 hours each
day, "making rounds and dressings daily at 9 a.m. and each evening
before 8 p.m." He was not allowed to examine female patients, "except
in the presence of a nurse," he could not "receive money or any other
remuneration from a patient or any visitor to the hospital," and he
was responsible for writing all of the case reports before a patient was
discharged.

Wesley Bourne, who had come to Montreal from Barbados to study medicine at McGill and who later became the first to apply the basic sciences to the practice of anesthesia, was called upon when needed to administer ether, chloroform, or nitrous oxide. John Cecil Lanthier was the hospital's first radiologist. He worked out of "a ground floor X-ray room that was little larger than a telephone booth." Lanthier recalled that when a doctor and his patient were both present in the room, he had "to crawl under the table to reach the X-ray control booth. The radiographic room and the darkroom were at loggerheads, certainly not on speaking terms. The situation was so hopeless that the darkroom insisted on moving into the stables, unheated and located in the far reaches of that vast estate, completely divorced and separate as to domicile."

Olive Fitzgibbon was named lady superintendent of the four secular graduate nurses and 16 nursing students. On August 16, 1924, St. Mary's Hospital (telephone number, WIlbank 5186) admitted as its first patient "a poor Irish domestic" who had toiled "longer than was good for her health." As the staff settled in, it quickly became apparent that the mansion was totally unsuited for use as a hospital. "It certainly aroused no pride in the Catholic community, in fact no real acceptance," Jack Dinan remarks in *St. Mary's Hospital: The Early Years*.

There were no service elevators in the building, which meant that patients had to be carried up and down staircases to the operating room on the second floor. There were four private suites and three public wards, but the building was infested with cockroaches and there were rats in the basement. "If you sat on the second floor at the nurses' desk, the rats would come out of the cupboard and look you straight in the eye," writes Dinan. Those who could afford to wouldn't go near the new hospital, even if had been Lord Shaughnessy's home.

During its first few years of operation, almost all of its patients were "the hopeless and neglected," indigents from the slums who "were not necessarily acceptable at other institutions." It was Fitzgibbon who almost singlehandedly built the hospital's reputation. "She gave the place a name not only through the care bestowed upon the patients but by the good training she imparted to the nurses," Emmett Mullally recorded in his diaries.

On May 16, 1924, the St. Mary's Hospital Ladies Auxiliary elected its first executive: seven vice presidents, 17 parish councillors, three conveners (membership, linens, and surgical dressings), a treasurer, a recording secretary, and a correspondence secretary. Two weeks later, Morrissey outlined her ambitious plans to the Auxiliary. She compared St. Mary's to St. Bernard's, a hospital in Chicago. "Its beginning was very humble, far more humble than St. Mary's, and its success was beyond all expectations," she said. Morrissey then spoke of her plans to build an addition to Shaughnessy House to accommodate her nursing school. Confident that a "training school will be opened shortly and will consist of 12 to 15 externes," she asked the women to raise money for blankets, sheets, and pillowcases. In order to keep expenses down, Morrissey added, "donations of preserves would also be welcome."

In a report filed with her superior in December, Morrissey mentions having raised $200,000 for her hospital and asks the nuns at Hôtel-Dieu to pray at Christmas for its success. "As you know, joy is transitory, and we have suffered a number of reversals and setbacks in our attempts to turn this historic house into a hospital…the names of St. Joseph and St. Thérèse are never invoked in vain."

Morrissey needed more than prayers to make ends meet. Within a year, her lack of administrative and people skills had become pitifully apparent. Nursing sisters brought in from convents in Kingston, Ontario, and Chatham and Campbellton, New Brunswick, to work with her didn't stay beyond their probationary period. Early records indicate a revolving door of religious staff. "She had a good appearance and on occasion was very pleasant," Hingston said of her. "She had a child-like faith, her religious life was beyond reproach. But," he observed, she was "inordinately vain and had poor judgment. She was not a good nurse, she neglected patients under her care, and was disliked by them. She was unforgiving."

Hints of even more trouble appeared in the hospital's first annual report, which was presented at a general meeting held on May 19, 1925: "The Medical Board feels acutely the lack of space in the hospital; the sisters have very crowded quarters, there is no room for an X-ray plant, and more space is essential to the efficiency of even a small first class hospital."

Housing for the nurses was found at 624 St. Marc Street, and the residence opened there on December 21, 1925. "The home leaves nothing to be desired." Fitzgibbon was pleased. "We have a charming living room, bright, airy class room, and bedrooms for 18 nurses."

Morrissey went out of her way to antagonize the new board president, Angus Robertson. Driven to distraction, he quit after six months, in November 1925, declaring that as long as Morrissey was running the place, "there was no possibility of success for the hospital." Donald Hingston took over as board president on November 17, and he exercised the patience of Job. "We dragged on," he said of the period. "No signs of enthusiasm anywhere, no signs of financial help and no desire to organize an appeal." In his dealings with Morrissey at the board level, Hingston adopted the only approach he could under the circumstances. He ignored her. "A resolution from the Board would be presented, I would ask for discussion. A tirade from Morrissey would follow, a vote would be taken, and I would cast the deciding ballot and the meeting would be over," Hingston lamented. In turn, Morrissey ignored the board. She had Birks, the city's most expensive jeweller, design and craft the pins that would be given to graduates at their capping ceremony without telling the board.

That decision would have far-reaching consequences and precipitate a clash of wills that would bring the hospital to its knees. "There could be a lot written about the pins for the nurses," Mullally wrote. "When brought to task by the Board for not consulting with Miss Fitzgibbon, who has given the place a name through the good training she has imparted to the nurses, Mother Morrissey persisted in her way of doing things. Dr. Hingston took the matter up, called a meeting of the directors, and had the pins designed and made up through the jewelry firm of Murray and O'Shea (who were interested in the hospital's progress). Mother Morrissey then informed the Board she would have nothing further to do with graduation exercises."

A fundraising campaign to cover the operating deficit and pay for X-ray machines was launched in 1926 with an objective of $75,000; it failed miserably, and the hospital could not afford to buy its own electrocardiograph machine. But, in spite of its internal problems, St. Mary's was fulfilling a need. During a typhoid epidemic in 1926, it treated more typhoid patients than any other hospital in the city; yet of the 130 typhoid deaths recorded that year, only one was reported at St. Mary's. "Anyone who was in a position to observe the unstinted manner in which Dr. Gaslin sacrificed himself during the epidemic will realize that there is a spirit in St. Mary's," the Knight News reported. "The care of typhoid patients is a great strain on a nursing staff, and through the ordeal there has been in evidence nothing but the completest cheerfulness and unlimited spirit of self sacrifice."

The first three nurses to complete their training at St. Mary's Hospital School of Nursing – Dorothy Donovan, Anne Lalonde, and Irene Nugent – received their diplomas on February 17, 1927. True to her word, Mother Morrissey boycotted the exercises held in the hospital chapel. Emmett Mullally wrote about the ceremony in his journal:

The night before the day of the graduation, Dr. Hingston did not know what form the ceremony might take as Mother Morrissey was quite peeved over not having her way. She wanted to hire a large hall and have speeches, etc. On the morning of the graduation Hingston sent word to the members of the Medical Board to be at the hospital at 3:45 p.m. to take part in the ceremony. The chapel was filled with friends and relatives, not merely of the graduates, but those interested in the hospital, and more people kept coming in. It was after four, the ceremony was to start, and no pins had arrived. The order for them had been given too late owing to the way Morrissey had acted. What was to be done?

Finally, at 4:30, Dr. Hingston presented each of the three with their diplomas in a purple soft leather cover, shakes hands with each and calls upon Dr. Devlin; Devlin under the disadvantage of little space and inappropriate setting makes a neat little talk which he can do very well…Father O'Reilly begins benediction, but before the benediction proper, the nurses read together a vow which in this instance was a translation from the French of a vow taken by nurses in a French hospital, another manifestation of Mother Morrissey's methods. At the conclusion of the benediction, the pins not yet arrived, we all went to the nurses' home where the three nurses were given three fine black leather bags. They cost $60 for the three and the cost was born by the five members of the Board: Hingston, Gray, Mullally, Mason and Wickham.

Having made all of the financial arrangements to buy the hospital with money she had raised herself, Mother Morrissey now took steps to seize absolute control. With the support of Father McDougald, the Redemptorist pastor of St. Ann's Parish, she moved to get rid of the hospital's lay board of directors and have St. Mary's placed under her jurisdiction. McDougald, an ascetic priest, wanted the hospital to be relocated to the poor Irish neighbourhood of Pointe-St-Charles, and he wanted the diocese to run it, with Mother Morrissey in charge. McDougald made his case to Bishop Gauthier. Gauthier ordered the board to turn the hospital over to Morrissey. Hingston refused.

A series of meetings was held between Hingston, Bishop Gauthier, McDougald, and Morrissey – "several of them very unpleasant," according to Hingston. What followed, he wrote with typical understatement, "was several more years of bickering and very unpleasant meetings." He continued, "Morrissey had now become impossible. She was determined to control the hospital personally. She purchased as she pleased, gave what orders she wished and co-operated with nobody." According to Hingston, she also displayed "an intense hatred" toward the head of the lay nurses, Miss Fitzgibbon. "Her constant rudeness to her was extraordinary and most uncalled for. Consequently, there was chaos in a small hospital." Minutes of the board meetings reveal that on several occasions, for reasons never made clear, Morrissey demanded that Fitzgibbon be fired. When the board refused, she insisted that her objections be inscribed in the official record. At one board meeting, she announced, "We protest, and wish this protest to be entered in the minutes; other means will be taken [to remove Fitzgibbon]. It will go before the public."

The hospital was losing money, and by 1929 it was $18,000 in debt. The first fundraising effort, mounted in January 1929, yielded less than $1,000. When the second group of nurses graduated, on February 8, Morrissey again refused to present the medals and diplomas. She also steadfastly refused to meet the mortgage payments, insisting that the hospital building was the board's responsibility, not hers. Her behaviour was now becoming a grave threat to the hospital's existence. Pushed along by Father McDougald, Morrissey offered to buy the hospital outright for her order of sisters, then she threatened to withdraw all nursing services unless the institution was handed over to her. "St. Mary's, still in its infancy, is nearing the close of its first five years of usefulness," she wrote. "We think the time is opportune to secure a site for a greater group of buildings, not only for hospital, outdoor department and nurses' home, but also for a community and novitiate where our sisters could complete their religious formation and qualify for the work for which it was originally planned."

Arrears on the building were growing. Morrissey wouldn't budge.

"The progress of the hospital has been retarded to a great extent by Mother Morrissey, the superioress," Mullally confided to his journal. "Although it was her insistence in keeping the idea of a hospital for the English-speaking Catholics before the public, and was responsible for the hospital being started, it is evident that she has not the requisite qualities for the head of such an institution; as a matter of fact, she possesses some qualities that are in a way desirable, yet she would not be offered as an example of the type of woman who make up the nursing religious orders."

It was obvious by now that Morrissey's ambition had exceeded her means. She had alienated every doctor, every nurse, and almost every donor. She had become, as Gauthier called her, "that harridan in a habit." For the good of all concerned, Hingston asked Gauthier to use his episcopal authority to silence Mother Morrissey. "You know her as well as I do," Gauthier countered. "Unless I lock her up in her room at St. Mary's such an order would be futile."

On September 10, Baroness Shaughnessy foreclosed on the mortgage. Bishop Gauthier met the directors in an emergency session on Friday, September 13. Hingston informed the directors that unless Gauthier used his episcopal authority to remove Mother Morrissey, "it would be useless to continue the work of the hospital. Liquidation and closure are the only alternative." Gauthier was not willing to fire Morrissey. There was, he said, absolutely nothing he could do to prevent her from opening a hospital on her own if she chose to do so. "She is brilliant, but antagonistic. If I were to order her to leave, she would go out on Dorchester Street, wave her arms about, and perhaps go over to the convent of the Little Sisters of the Poor as she has threatened to do. Serious scandal must be avoided at all costs." If he silenced her, he continued, "her fledgling order might claim it was being oppressed, cause bitter feeling," and take the matter over his head to Rome. But Gauthier did agree to talk to Morrissey again to see whether he could persuade her to change her mind. He was unable to sway her. He telephoned Hingston at 8:30 on Sunday morning, September 15. "It is all here, this is the end of St. Mary's," Gauthier said. The Hospitalières would assume the mortgage on the building only if the board cancelled the St. Mary's charter and turned the hospital over to them so in due course the nuns might apply for their own charter. Hingston was having none of it. "As there was nothing else we could do but hold to our principles, we gave orders for the hospital to be closed," he wrote in his memoirs.

On October 8, 1929, St. Mary's Hospital, "bankrupt, financially and emotionally," shut its doors. A group of 18 of the hospital's doctors signed an affidavit in support of Hingston's decision. "The financial condition of St. Mary's does not warrant its continued operation," the affidavit read, "and especially whereas there is lack of union between the elements of the directorate which cannot be remedied, it is resolved with deep regret, to close the hospital." Two weeks later, the stock market crashed. It was the beginning of the Great Depression, and it seemed that St. Mary's would never reopen.

Patients were farmed out to other hospitals, the secular nurses found work at the Royal Victoria Hospital, and Mother Morrissey went back to Hôtel-Dieu, where she was instrumental in starting the hospital museum. She later took much of the credit for a biography of Hôtel-Dieu founder Jeanne Mance, which had in fact been written by Joseph Foran.

"She was a great general, but only an army of penitent saints could work with her," maintains Jack Dinan. "She was misunderstood by the medical group in spite of warnings by the Bishop....She was a bred-in-the-convent, devoted and dedicated Hospitalière of St-Joseph... wholly absorbed with the idea of organizing an English chapter of the Hospitalières in Montreal, staffing it with nursing sisters and running it as any Hôtel-Dieu in Québec was run. It was not within her experience nor her convictions to accept the idea of lay control, and she was therefore bitterly disillusioned when the medical board employed a lay nursing supervisor to teach her nurses. She never recovered from what she considered to be an affront to her."

CHAPTER TWO

A hospital dedicated to the most sacred of mothers cannot be allowed
to fail.... Where buildings are erected in Mary's name, all are home and no
one is a stranger.... Mary is our mother. To be part of this place is to be part
of a family that reveres her name.... No institution that bears her name
can be allowed to fail.
~ Sister St. Simon (Victoire Séguin)

Hingston refused to be defeated.

Encouraged by Wilfrid Emmett McDonagh, the founding pastor of
the Ascension of Our Lord Parish in Westmount, Hingston mobilized
his own resources. The same week the hospital closed, he went to
Quebec City to ask Premier Louis-Alexandre Taschereau and the provincial secretary, Louis-Athanase David, to help him salvage the hospital.
Hingston was able to argue that during the five years St. Mary's had been
open it had become indispensable: 4,363 in-patients and 2,000 outpatients had been treated, and 1,827 operations had been performed.

Taschereau offered $50,000 to refinance the hospital, provided that
a community of nursing sisters could be found who were willing to
keep it open. Hingston then paid a visit to the Sisters of Providence
of St. Vincent de Paul – a Montreal order founded in 1844 by Émilie
Tavernier-Gamelin – but the tone of the meeting was "quite cool. The
sisters at once came to the point and asked in whom the ownership
would be invested," he tells us. "When I said it would be in the corporation of directors and not in the sisterhood, they refused." Then,
on New Year's Day, 1930, Hingston went to see one of his mother's
influential friends, Mother Margaret McKenna, who had for years
been the bursar for the Sisters of Charity of Montreal, more com-
monly known as the Grey Nuns. Everyone in Montreal knew "Mother

McKenna of the Grey Nuns." She had grown up in the village of Côte-des-Neiges, where her father had a florist business. She had started an orphanage, founded a veterans' hospital, and successfully lobbied to have Parliament Square in Old Montreal renamed Place d'Youville in honour of Marguerite d'Youville, the nun who founded the Sisters of Charity in 1755.

Hingston found McKenna ill, and not very encouraging. The Grey Nuns, she told him, had overextended themselves by opening hospitals in Western Canada and the United States. If they were to accept his offer to run St. Mary's, she said, they would have to close one of those hospitals. McKenna also "very naturally hesitated about putting [the Grey Nuns] in a position largely dependent on laymen." The following week, however, she had a change of heart and informed Hingston that, "after much agonizing," the Grey Nuns had decided that they would close their hospital in Nashua, New Hampshire, so that they could keep St. Mary's open. A contract initialled on February 13 by Hingston and the Grey Nuns' superior general, Mother Marie-Louise-Octavie Dugas, gave the nuns absolute control of the nursing school and staff.

According to the terms of the three-page contract, the Grey Nuns "may engage [nurses], fix their remuneration and discharge them.... The visiting of the sick shall be under the control and supervision of the sisters, who may determine the days and hours on which such visits may be made, and the visitors who may be allowed or refused admission." In addition, St. Mary's Hospital would pay each nursing sister $200 per year and assume "all of the expenses connected with the administration and maintenance of the School of Nursing." Article 2, the most important clause, which would later prove to be the most contentious, gave the Grey Nuns the authority to "purchase all provisions, foods, linen, bedding, ordinary furnishings, etc. for the sick."

Victoire Séguin, who went by the name of Sister St. Simon, was brought in from Calgary to be superintendent of nurses. She was a strict but serene 51-year-old nun who had completed graduate studies in pharmacy in Toledo, Ohio, and, after working in a number of

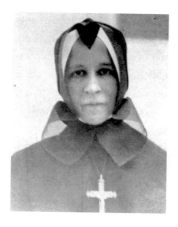

Sister St. Simon.
"A hospital dedicated to Mary cannot
be allowed to fail."

hospitals in the Maritimes and New England, had been named
superior of Calgary's Holy Cross Hospital in 1929. The third child in
a family of 12 children, Séguin was originally from Stoney Point,
Ontario, but she was raised in Windsor and Detroit. She entered the
Grey Nuns in 1900, taking her vows in 1908. Shortly after moving to
Calgary, she had undergone a mastoid operation, which had left her
face partially paralyzed. In a letter to Hingston, Séguin explained why
she was so eager to come to Montreal. "A hospital dedicated to the
most sacred of mothers cannot be allowed to fail. When the Virgin
Mary becomes the patron of a cause, she will never abandon it. Where
buildings are erected in Mary's name, all are home and no one is a
stranger. As superior I will consecrate myself to suffering and be an
example to those who lead a religious life. On this point I am more
and more adamant."

With Sister St. Simon in charge, the Grey Nuns moved in on March 1,
and St. Mary's reopened on March 19, 1930, the patronal feast day of
St. Joseph, Canada's patron saint. The following day, the first patient
was admitted, a woman named Mary Boyle.

Hingston then launched a fundraising campaign and out of his
own pocket paid $8,000 to professional consultant Sam Stalford of

Toronto to run the campaign. Hingston's efforts, essentially unsupported by his colleagues, were underwritten by his mother, Lady Hingston. Stalford concluded that it would cost $4,000 a bed to build a new hospital and $1,000 a bed each year after that to maintain it. Therefore, if it was to be a 200-bed hospital, at least $1 million had to be amassed. Their objective was spelled out: If the city's 18 English-speaking Roman Catholic parishes could among them come up with $250,000 to kick-start the campaign, then the City of Montreal would contribute $100,000, and the board could depend on a matching grant from the province of $400,000. The remaining $250,000, known as the "Citizen's Objective," would be raised by targeting a small group of rich corporate donors through a "special names committee." Targets for each of the parishes were established: St. Patrick's, Ascension of Our Lord, St. Michael's, St. Augustine's of Canterbury, and St. Willibrord's would each be expected to raise $10,000; St. Anthony's and St. Raphael's, $6,000 each; the poorer parishes, such as St. Ann's, St. Agnes's, St. Dominic's, Holy Family, St. Thomas Aquinas's, St. Aloysius's, and St. Ignatius's, $4,000 each; and St. Brendan's, St. Mary's, and Holy Cross, among the smallest parishes, $1,000 each.

A survey of the parishes revealed a mixed reaction. Hingston was "very discourteously received," by Holy Family's pastor, Aloysius Walls, who accused him of "grandiose ambitions" that were "too much for a struggling Irish community to support." If a hospital was to be built, Walls complained, the proper procedure was for the Bishop, not Hingston, to poll the priests. Father Thomas Francis Heffernan at St. Augustine's of Canterbury wanted nothing to do with the project if French-speaking nuns were involved. Gerald McShane at St. Patrick's imperiously dismissed Hingston, telling him that as far as his parishioners were concerned, "the appeal for St. Mary's is dead." Reverend Philip Brady, one of Mother Morrissey's camp followers and pastor at St. Mary's, told Hingston that he would not support a fundraising campaign unless Morrissey was involved. Aware that he might be perceived as a liability, Hingston was prepared to step down as chairman of the hospital board. He tried to persuade one of his cronies, Lieutenant Colonel William Patrick O'Brien, a prominent broker, to take charge.

"As O'Brien was a very rich man, he could make a much greater success of the venture than I could," Hingston wrote. "I suggested that he make the building of St. Mary's the magnum opus of his life. I told him I would retire, give him the chair, and he would be known as the founder of the hospital." But O'Brien was involved in organizing the Federation of Catholic Charities to help those on the dole during the Depression, and he dismissed the hospital project as impractical. In fact, he recommended that St. Mary's be "closed and that no further financial obligations assumed in its operation."

For the hospital to succeed, it had to have the wholehearted co-operation of every parish in the city. What Hingston desperately needed was a pastoral letter from Bishop Gauthier throwing the full weight of the archdiocese behind the project. "We know Your Grace's worry and anxiety," Hingston wrote to Bishop Gauthier on February 21, "but we assure Your Grace that in years to come you will never have reason to regret the help." Gauthier ignored the letter. An episcopal endorsement seemed unlikely.

Then a new voice was heard. Luke Callaghan, the pastor of St. Michael's Parish in Mile End, was well connected to the offices of the archdiocese – so well, in fact, that in 1904 he became the first priest to preach in English at Notre-Dame Basilica. He had also been vice chancellor of the archbishop's palace when Gauthier was still an underling. On August 29, Callaghan called on Hingston and said that he, Hingston, should draft the pastoral letter he so urgently required. Callaghan would present it to Gauthier. So Hingston wrote: "St. Mary's Hospital, with a humble beginning and under the most trying handicaps, has performed a splendid service to our people and to the citizens of Montreal. I realize there is a great need for a larger and more modern hospital such as the present Board of Directors of St. Mary's now proposes to build. Their campaign, therefore, with the object of raising the necessary funds, meets with my warmest approval and blessing, and I commend it to our people in the hope that they will contribute most generously to our worthy cause." To Hingston's amazement, Callaghan returned with the letter bearing the Bishop's signature within the hour. "Until that moment Gauthier had never shown himself friendly to the enterprise," Hingston wrote in his memoir. "In my opinion, Luke Callaghan saved St. Mary's."

A more formal pastoral letter was read in the parishes on Sunday, September 7. In it, the bishop declared that "raising a sum of money sufficient to build a new, thoroughly modern and fire proof hospital" met with his approval, and he urged all Catholics "to recognize their duty to the sick and afflicted by a generous response to this appeal." No Catholic, not even McShane, could ignore that directive.

Motivated by the new developments, the Ladies Auxiliary held an "at-home benefit" at the Mount Royal Hotel on October 21, at which they raised $5,000. A financial plan was drawn up: English-speaking Catholics were expected to provide $250,000; corporate sponsors would chip in $300,000; the province, $350,000; and the City of Montreal, $100,000. On October 29, 1930, Hingston wrote to Mayor Camillien Houde asking for a municipal grant. "It is a well known fact that the City of Montreal can do with more hospital beds and while St. Mary's Hospital has been doing its share in a small way, towards providing medical care and treatment for our citizens, it would be a tragedy to permit the present small hospital with such a splendid record of service behind it to go out of existence for the [lack] of financial aid."

Then Hingston asked 18 of the city's English-speaking pastors to meet with him on November 24. He convinced them to pledge the "moral support, co-operation and financial assistance" of their respective congregations. "For the first time a large number of our pastors sat down together," he wrote. "The jarring element had been excluded. Everyone enjoyed himself thoroughly." Conspicuous by their absence were the pastors of the parishes of St. Patrick's, St. Ann's, and

Holy Family; but they had no choice but to fall in line. There were, however, some irritating setbacks. Fundraising was postponed for six months to permit O'Brien and the newly established Federation of Catholic Charities to meet the $75,000 objective of the federation's first campaign.

"In all my experience in directing fund raising campaigns I have never before been faced with circumstances that have continuously arisen, none of which have offered anything in the way of constructive progress," fundraising campaign head Stalford wrote to the board. "The true facts of the case are that the English Speaking Catholics of Montreal, as a whole, recognize the need for and the majority desire to have a new modern up to date hospital. But the different groups apparently interested appear to have such a difference of opinion that it is impossible to proceed with any definite plan until one of these groups assumes responsibility of proceeding with the project. It means we have to stop procrastinating…and face the situation with a determination to carry out the original plans for the campaign and bring it to a successful conclusion."

The setbacks were temporary. On February 9, 1931, Montreal's Executive Committee not only approved Hingston's request for a grant but also substantially increased it. Thanks largely to lobbying by Alderman Tom O'Connell, the city agreed to assume one-third of the cost of the proposed million-dollar building. "It is very rarely that a deputation when asking for grants from the city receives more than it requests," observed the *Montreal Star*. "This precedent was created today."

On Sunday, March 15, a cardboard model of the hospital building was driven through the city streets as part of the annual St. Patrick's Day parade. Artists went to work designing a hospital crest featuring "a bust reproduction of the Blessed Virgin on the junction of a red cross, surrounded by a scroll." On May 11, 1931, the general appeal for $1 million was launched, with each parish asked to "make its contribution in cash." The drive raised $360,465.93. "In all my experience in conducting campaigns this appeal was the most difficult I have ever attempted because every known element and circumstance confronted us," Stalford wrote. "In ordinary times the same effort would have resulted in securing over two million dollars."

At a board meeting held in April 1932, it was decreed that for the "purposes of preserving continuity," the old hospital would remain open until a new one was built, "even though operating conditions are unfavourable and likely to so continue until the new hospital can receive patients." At the same board meeting, it was explained to members that a hospital building was being designed "along lines that will permit extension and development as time and conditions warrant," and a discussion was undertaken to determine where the hospital should be built. Some thought that it should be located near the campus of Loyola College in Notre-Dame-de-Grâce, others, somewhere in Pointe-St-Charles. Many of the sites Hingston had considered ideal now seemed, upon further reflection, "too small, too far away, or too expensive." It was Mother McKenna who suggested seven *arpents* of land (281,000 square feet) in Côte-des-Neiges, the village where she had been raised. The site was in the shadow of St. Joseph's Oratory, directly behind Collège Notre-Dame. The property had been set aside as farmland by the Sulpicians in 1698. Its most recent owner, François-Xavier Cardinal, had died, and his widow had put the family farm up for sale. As soon as Hingston expressed interest in the property, however, the local ward-heeling alderman, Pierre Deguire, tried to block the sale. Deguire, as it turned out, was the front man for Reverend Alfred Nantel, the parish priest who had built his presbytery and a mission church, St. Thomas à Becket, next door to the proposed site. Nantel wanted the Cardinal property for his parish. He planned to buy it, subdivide it for residential use, and use the profits from the real estate sales to finance the building of a church. However, Mother McKenna's brother, Leo McKenna, persuaded Deguire that it was not in Father Nantel's best interests to oppose construction of the hospital. To reinforce his point, McKenna later ran for city council in the district and made the construction of the hospital the single issue of

his campaign. He won, served on city council for 20 years, and remained a loyal hospital champion until his death in 1956.

According to the deed of sale, the Board of Directors paid $45,840
for the property. Hingston wanted Boston architects Edward Stevens
and Frederick Lee to design St. Mary's. The pair had been responsible
for Hôpital Notre-Dame, which had opened in 1922. But, experienc-
ing chest pains and suffering from a heart disorder undoubtedly
brought on by the stress he had been under for the previous three
years or so, Hingston resigned as chairman of the board on May 26,
1931. He was succeeded by Senator Wilfrid Laurier McDougald, who
insisted on a Quebec-based team of architects and put his personal
secretary, Aloysius Chopin, in charge of the project. Edward J. Turcotte
and John Archibald were hired. "There was much trouble and many
discussions over the plans, tenders and contracts," Hingston recalled.
"I broke down with an attack of myocarditis and for some months
could take no active part in the planning which went ahead with – I
fear many mistakes. However, we muddled through." John Quinlan,
who had submitted a tender of $553,880, was engaged as the building's
general contractor, and James Ballantyne was paid $159,113 to install
plumbing, heating, and ventilation. Since the city was footing a third
of the cost, a restriction was imposed: "In making all purchases, con-
tractors shall give preference to those materials made in Montreal or
elsewhere in the Province of Quebec." The board made it clear that
"No changes of any kind should be authorized after construction
starts...and that the architects and engineers will be held morally
responsible to see that the program is carried out."

Sod was turned on Tuesday, May 23, 1933. "To keep a lid on costs
workers were paid 15 cents an hour, less than the minimum wage. The
Montreal Star condemned the exploitation in its editorial pages. While
it acknowledges that the practice was widespread during the Depression, the newspaper denounced the low wages 'as a retrograde step, a
setback in the centuries old campaign for a square deal for labour.'"

Stung by the media criticism, the board wrote to John Quinlan on

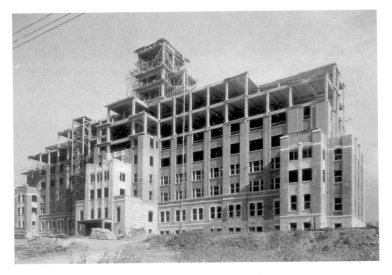

St. Mary's under construction, spring 1934.
Courtesy of Dr. Richard Moralejo.

July 6 expressing its "embarrassment" over the wages he was paying his workmen. In one isolated incident, the workers walked off the job for three days to protest their low rate of pay, but the matter was quickly resolved, and construction of "Montreal's newest palace of healing," as the newspapers now called it, continued ahead of schedule. The hospital rose quickly. Steel work was completed by March, the frame was enclosed by the end of the summer, and general finishing work was done in three months. Chief porter Roger Kelly, a recent Irish immigrant from Galway, was the first to report for duty in the new building, assuming responsibility for the security of stores and supervising installation of the new hospital's equipment. St. Mary's Memorial Hospital opened on November 24, 16 months after the sod-turning.

The *Gazette* reported the ambulance transfer of 20 patients from the old building to the new one. "In order to facilitate the difficult task, all convalescents sufficiently recovered were discharged, which left only 20 for removal," the newspaper noted. The Shaughnessy House

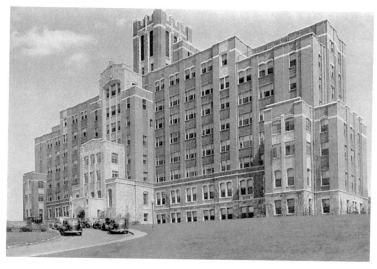

Montreal's newest "Palace of Healing," 1938.
Photo by Graetz Bros.

hospital was sold for $40,000 to the Sisters of Service, who turned it into a home for unwed mothers. The new hospital, like the old, allowed patients to draw upon the comforts of their Roman Catholic faith in their suffering, and it strived to respect the dignity of all patients, regardless of religious affiliation.

Accommodation for student nurses was found in a building across the street from the hospital, 3835 Lacombe Avenue, which the hospital planned to lease until a permanent nurses' residence could be built. Reverend Thomas O'Reilly, "a quiet, almost invisible man, who brought unobtrusive comfort to the sick," became St. Mary's first resident chaplain. There were 11 staff doctors and another 60 physicians and surgeons with hospital privileges. "What we brought to the new hospital was a sense of family. Not only did this sense of family remain, it was soon extended to the new people who joined us. It was a happy, home-like atmosphere to work in," Jack Dinan recalled.

Sir Henry Gray, a burly Aberdeen Scot, arrived by default in 1935 and added a great deal of cachet to the institution. Gray had served with distinction in the Boer War and the First World War. Knighted for his work as a surgeon with the Third British Army in France during the First World War, he was considered "the last of the god-like temperamental surgeons." Gray had, in fact, been recruited to come to Montreal as surgeon-in-chief for the Royal Victoria Hospital, but because the Royal Victoria's president, Sir Vincent Meredith, had made the appointment without seeking the approval of his medical board, bureaucratic noses were put out of joint, and shortly after Gray arrived he was forced to relinquish the position. He went into private practice and acquired hospital privileges at St. Mary's. Gray brought with him to St. Mary's his medical assistant, Frank Scully, a "short, humorous and handsome" doctor who was impossible to dislike, "even when you knew he was making a patsy out of you." Gray is remembered as being one of the first doctors who encouraged his patients to get out of bed within days of surgery at a time when the general practice was to keep those who had undergone surgery in bed for at least a week.

Hingston became the hospital's first surgeon-in-chief, and thereafter, until the day he died, he was revered by all and fondly referred to as "the Chief."

Lieutenant Colonel Charles Peters, a native of St. John's, Newfoundland, who had graduated from McGill in medicine with first-class honours in 1898, and who, like Gray, had fought in both the Boer War and the First World War, was brought in from the Montreal General to set up the Department of Medicine. Peters, a superb diagnostician and teacher, was highly regarded by interns. However, he left St. Mary's within the year, and Leo Mason, who had furthered his education at Hôpital Laennec in Paris and at the Mayo Clinic, replaced him.

Norman Williamson, who still looked like the football player he had once been, was a naturally assertive redhead with a "roaring, whirling type of personality"; he took over the still new and limited specialty of orthopedics, initiating improved care for musculoskeletal disorders. "Mac" McGovern, one of the hospital's original hardworking founders, headed the Department of Dermatology.

Dr. A.G. "Bert" McAuley was put in charge of the Department of Ophthalmology, which was being influenced by new developments in the aeronautical industry. Neurologist Thomas Hoen, a native of Baltimore who had moved to Montreal to study with Wilder Penfield, was named chief of the Department of Neurosurgery. There he worked with Arthur Wilson Young, a neurologist from Revelstoke, British Columbia, who had won the Holmes Medal upon graduating from McGill in 1921 and who had gone on to study psychiatry in Boston, London, Paris, and Berlin. Ansel Tanney came from Western Hospital to open the Department of Genitourinary Medicine, and James Rogers was engaged to head the Department of Otolaryngology. James MacIntyre, who was originally from Cape Breton and who had worked for the Price Brothers paper company in Trois-Rivières, was hired as the hospital's chief maintenance engineer, and he kept things running for decades to come.

The new hospital was short on medical specialists and long on general practitioners, so accredited staff members of the Royal Victoria and the Montreal General were offered admitting privileges and welcomed as consultants. St. Mary's quickly established a reputation as a first-rate, "high intensity" maternity hospital. Initially, obstetrics and gynecology were separate departments, with James Goodall – handsome, dapper, and dashing – brought in from the Royal Victoria to be chief of Gynecology, and Dunstan Gray – no relation to Sir Henry – appointed as chief of Obstetrics. Gray, a McGill graduate, had completed his postgraduate studies in Paris. He was a kindly man, a skilled physician, and a considerate administrator. He pioneered the use of "small quantities of a minimally toxic and a dependable drug," sodium pentothal, to reduce labour pains. Under his direction, the Department of Obstetrics became a showcase, with private and semi-private rooms, two state-of-the-art delivery theatres with adjoining labour rooms, a 25-crib nursery, and a separate isolation area with observation windows so that relatives could view the babies. The department's senior obstetrician and gynecologist, Richard M.H. Power, was an excellent doctor, if somewhat feisty and overbearing, who had been

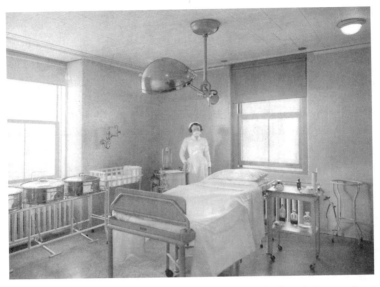

The maternity room, 1935, was busy from the day the hospital opened.

on staff since 1926. He devised a unique surgical practice known around the hospital as the "Power twist." He would apply a short cotton drain to a wound, fold it, and, as he inserted it, give it a theatrical twist. Later, he'd pluck it out with similar flair and assure the patient that the wound was healing well. Such minor theatrics did no harm, but no other doctor believed that it did the patient any good.

This fact is now largely forgotten, but it is worth mentioning here. In the mid-1930s, giving birth and being born were dangerous things: one in every 150 pregnancies resulted in the death of the mother; and each year, 15,000 Quebec babies died before they were three months old. Gray established firm rules about who could and who could not perform deliveries, what steps had to be followed, and when Caesarean sections were allowed. He developed the department and staffed it with first-rate nurses, interns, and residents. Gertrude G. Pearson, who came from Sherbrooke, Quebec, and who had obtained her medical degree from McGill in 1933, was hired as a clinical assistant, becoming the first female doctor on staff. The standards at St. Mary's were so high that the hospital began attracting maternity patients from the Royal Victoria and the Montreal General. Under the direction of Dr. Basil Cuddihy, the Knights of Columbus ran the hospital's blood donor clinic, and Dr. James Goodall inaugurated a placental blood bank, which he boasted was "one of the greatest advances in the history of modern medicine." Goodall had started saving placental blood from normal deliveries, which otherwise would have been flushed away. He sealed it in flasks for 90 days and used it for transfusions. The approach was so innovative that St. Mary's could brag that "the technique originating in the research laboratory of this hospital is being adopted by a large number of well known hospitals in America and abroad."

Jack Gerrie, one of the country's first qualified plastic surgeons, came aboard as a consultant in 1935. A native of Stratford, Ontario, Gerrie had graduated in dentistry from the University of Alberta in Edmonton when he was 21 years old and received his medical degree from McGill in 1931. This pioneer in the emerging field of reconstructive surgery went on to work at St. Bartholomew's Hospital in London with Archibald McIndoe and McIndoe's cousin, Sir Harold Gillies, the doyens of plastic surgery, both of whom were later knighted for their work. Gerrie also studied otolaryngology at London's Hospital in Golden Square and eventually became a leading expert in facial surgery, a professor at McGill University, and president of the American Society of Maxillofacial Surgeons.

St. Mary's was a money-losing proposition from the moment it opened. The first annual report, delivered in the boardroom of the new building on May 16, 1935, indicated that the hospital was losing $6,000 a month – "far above the estimated $45,000 a year calculated when the hospital opened."

Even after the Depression, large numbers of people couldn't afford to pay their hospital bills, and many went into debt. Initially, except for maternity cases, Irish Catholics were reluctant to use the new hospital. Although the public wards were filled, the more expensive semi-private and private rooms often sat empty. For many, the hospital was either too expensive or too far off the beaten path. During the first year of operation, St. Mary's treated a mere 2,754 patients, 95 percent of them ward cases from Verdun, Griffintown, and Pointe-St-Charles. Of these, 75 percent were Roman Catholic, 23 percent were Protestant, and one percent were Hebrew. The Department of Obstetrics, which delivered 283 babies that first year, was the busiest. A total of 846 surgical operations were performed that year. The overall occupancy rate was less than 40 percent, which permitted 63 student nurses to move into rooms on the seventh floor that had been meant for patients. Dunstan Gray didn't like the situation. There were more nuns and nurses living in the building than patients. He recommended spending $175,000 to build "a cheap nursing home" and opening the seventh floor to patients. His recommendation was ignored. Gray was battling public opinion, which at the time frowned upon women working outside the home. During the Depression, women were not supposed to deprive men of their jobs and thus rob them of the dignity their role as breadwinners afforded them. Gerald McShane put it in more homely terms when speaking to a graduating class, suggesting to the women about to be capped that nursing was not their true vocation. "Marriage is the true vocation of every Catholic girl," he insisted, "and a girl could receive no better training for becoming a wife than the training she received as a nurse." McShane urged them to be inspired by St. Mary's Hospital itself, "which stands high on a hill top and brings sunshine into the lives of hundreds of people daily."

In June 1936, Sister St. Simon left to become superior of a hospital in Biggar, Saskatchewan; she was replaced by Sister Mary-Ann Casey, originally from New Brunswick, who had been superior of the Grey Nuns in Alberta. At the same time, another of Hingston's cronies, Major Daniel O'Donahoe, a career soldier from Brockville, Ontario, succeeded Taggart Smyth as board president. O'Donahoe had been staff officer with the Fourth Canadian Division during the First World War and was twice mentioned in dispatches and awarded the Croix de guerre and the Distinguished Service Order for gallantry. After the war, he moved to Montreal, where he became general manager of the Canadian Industrial Alcohol Company and was actively involved with the Federation of Catholic Charities.

St. Mary's opened its Department of Dentistry in April 1937 in a four-foot-square room that had been used to store plaster. "In that space we had a dental cabinet, a chair so rusty it refused to adjust and a drill that worked only after proper coaxing," recalled John Dohan, the flinty dentist who set up the department. "Plaster casts were put on and taken off at the same time that dental patients were treated." Dohan, like Dr. McGovern, came from Danville, Quebec. He was educated at Bishop's University's medical school and at McGill University, and he had served in the First World War with the 55th Irish Rangers as a company commander. He had practised dentistry in Trois-Rivières and Grand-Mère before marrying into a monied Montreal family. His wife, Juliette Timmins, was a daughter of mining magnate Noah Anthony Timmins, who discovered gold in Cobalt, Ontario, in 1910 and who became one of the hospital's most generous benefactors. Dohan was one of the original founders of the Mount Stephen Club, on Drummond Street, which opened in 1926. A hard-nosed, rigid man, he remained at St. Mary's until 1949, when he left to teach prosthodontics at McGill; he would later become the first Canadian to be elected president of the American Academy of Restorative Dentistry.

The staff began to grow rapidly. Arthur Wilson Young, the neurologist from British Columbia, numbered among the new faces. His fellow McGill graduate John Lanthier, by now "the best diagnostic reader of the abdominal flat plate in Montreal," came from the Royal Victoria Hospital to run the Department of Radiology. Obstetrician Louis James Quinn, a 1936 McGill graduate, began at St. Mary's as an intern. Other specialists with promising futures who worked on staff either full- or part-time included: Mario Orlando, engaged as a junior clinical assistant in surgery; Raymond Hughes, who would set up the rheumatology clinic; Joe Pritchard, a pathologist; and Neil Feeney, a cardiologist from the Montreal General Hospital.

Because of its improved status, St. Mary's was reclassified by the Quebec government as a class A institution. In theory, this meant that the government per diem rate for patients would increase from $1.34 to $2 a day, but the hospital had trouble collecting, and the board's anxiety over finances continued to mount. To raise money, the board authorized the printing of a souvenir booklet, "subject to strict censorship in regard to the printed matter," which sold for 25 cents.

The Ladies Auxiliary continued to be active fundraisers. On October 29, 1937, its first fundraising ball, billed as a "Gay Gambol," was held at the Mount Royal Hotel. More than 700 guests danced to the music of the Maurice Davis Orchestra. The ball raised over $700, and, until 1973, it remained a formal, white-tie affair on the city's social calendar.

Lady Tweedsmuir, the wife of Canada's governor general, toured the hospital on November 26. Especially impressed by the maternity ward, she encouraged the Ladies Auxiliary to start a maternity committee to provide layettes and milk to impoverished women who could not afford clothing for their infants. This inspired Hingston's daughter, Katherine Gallery, to establish the St. Mary's Hospital Maternity Committee. The senior group advised the members of Gallery's junior group to "content themselves with being groundskeepers, taking an interest in flowers, decorations in public wards, and help with the annual dance." But the junior group had greater ambitions, and soon a rivalry between the two organizations surfaced. The friction between them would persist for years.

The attention they received in the society pages raised morale, but it didn't help to raise cash for the hospital. In its first four years in the new building, St. Mary's had run up a $65,000 deficit, and the future looked grim. In April 1938, a campaign to raise $500,000 to add a west wing to the main building was announced, but it proved to be a pipe dream. The board then looked to the federal government for assistance. The Department of Veterans Affairs in Ottawa had begun acquiring land for a veterans' hospital west of St. Mary's, with an option to develop property next to St. Mary's between Lacombe Avenue and Jean-Brillant Street. The board president, Major O'Donahoe, had an innovative idea to upgrade the mission of the hospital. He thought that it would make more sense for the federal government to build wings to St. Mary's that could accommodate veterans than to spend money upgrading the Nazareth Institute, a federal chronic care hospital, for that purpose. O'Donahoe wrote to the minister in charge and assured him that the proposed St. Mary's wings "would be under the direction of the Department of Pensions and Health, and later would become part of the [hospital] to which they have been added." The federal government, however, had already contracted other Montreal hospitals to provide medical services for veterans, including the Royal Victoria and the Montreal General. O'Donahoe's idea was never even considered.

CHAPTER THREE

Once the Christian motive of charity is removed, a civic hospital becomes just another institution where bureaucracy reigns and the patient is reduced to a number.
~ Aloysius Chopin

The Second World War, which began in September 1939, took a heavy toll in terms of money, material, and personnel at St. Mary's, and it disrupted the hospital's established routine. Each day, the board was confronted with "a steady increase in the work of the hospital, a natural consequence of growth, and departments at times which were actually overworked." Everything was in short supply except government red tape.

The immediate impact was felt in the obstetrics and pediatrics departments. During the war years, an estimated 500,000 "goodbye babies" were born in Canada – 7,500 of them at St. Mary's. In 1938, there had been 541 deliveries; that jumped 26 percent in the first year of the war, and by war's end, deliveries at St. Mary's had increased by 111 percent. In January 1941, the St. Mary's Hospital Maternity Committee started inscribing the names of every infant born in the hospital in a gold birthday book, a tradition that continued until 1988. Guest books were left outside the delivery room, and anxious fathers-to-be were encouraged to scribble their thoughts in them as they waited for their wives to give birth. Among the more clever jottings were:

> All night and day, doc did you call,
> I rush to the nursery, its mine after all!
> Pressed to the glass, my eyes search in vain,
> I think I've been gypped.
> They all look the same!

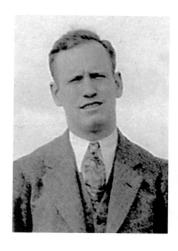

Dr. Gerald Altimas, father of the
Department of Obstetrics and Gynecology.

And:

> Here I write with pride and joy,
> For today we got a baby boy!
> The joy is shared by yet another,
> Now that Lisa has a baby brother!

Sportswriter Patrick Curran, waiting for the birth of his child, wondered:

> Will it be a boy or girl?
> What will be the name?
> As long as they are both healthy,
> Isn't it all the same?

Since the country needed many soldiers in a hurry, 30 members of St. Mary's administrative, medical, nursing, and maintenance teams left to fight. Among them were: Jack Dinan, then 33, who had just completed his postgraduate studies in surgery in London; John Emmett Donahoe, a 29-year-old doctor from Rocanville, Saskatchewan, who had recently graduated from Dalhousie University's medical school;

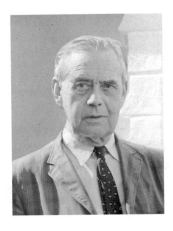

Dr. Harold Dolan, Hingston's son-in-law, ran the hospital during the Second World War.

John, "Mac" McGovern's 27-year-old son, just out of McGill; the hospital's superintendent, Aloysius Chopin, who joined the Royal Canadian Air Force; and Charles Pick, who had been an intern for less than six months. Board chairman Major O'Donahoe was transferred to defence headquarters in Ottawa; he was replaced by James A. Kennedy.

By 1941, the Board of Directors had been informed that some hospital departments were overburdened, and "accommodation" was "lamentably inadequate. The Obstetrics Department in particular is compelled to occupy the whole of the 4th floor, and the Department of Pediatrics is already too small."

At that time, the Quebec government controlled all social agencies through the Church. Alex Carter, a highly qualified administrator who had just completed his graduate studies in canon law in Rome, moved into the chaplain's quarters, where he would remain until 1958, when he was appointed bishop of Sault Ste. Marie, Ontario.

In June 1941, Lawrence Whelan was consecrated as Montreal's first English-speaking bishop, and he was automatically named honorary board chairman, a position he held for the next 20 years. At the board's request, Dr. Harold Sylvester Dolan stepped in to manage the hospital while Chopin was overseas. Dolan was married to Donald Hingston's daughter, Andrea. A gentle, hardworking surgeon "with good hands and a fine technique," Dolan had come to Montreal from New Brunswick, where his father ran a lumber mill. Dolan had obtained an arts degree from St. Francis Xavier University before completing a degree in medicine at Dalhousie in 1923. He joined St. Mary's in 1928 only because, as a Roman Catholic, he had not been accepted as a resident at the Royal Victoria Hospital. Although Dolan was Hingston's son-in-law, the two rarely socialized. Hingston, it seems, thought Dolan was too old for his daughter and didn't come from a similar patrician background. Hingston may have also resented the fact that, by all accounts, Dolan was the better surgeon. In addition to his role at the hospital, Dolan had also taken on the position of senior medical officer in charge of the Royal Canadian Army Medical Corps reserves in Montreal.

Dolan had little taste for administration, and during the 1941 annual general meeting told the board as much. "Great War Number Two, in which our country is so actively engaged, has reduced not only the profession of doctors and nurses, but has created a difficulty of readily securing skilled and unskilled workers in practically every department of the hospital; our staff of intern doctors was disrupted more than once during the year by the enlistment of some of its members for overseas." As it had become more and more expensive to run St. Mary's, Dolan recommended that the hospital hire a competent full-time manager who could keep expenses in line and take absolute control over the hospital's finances. The board concurred, and it had the good sense to hire as superintendent Colonel John Brannen, who had just retired as Quebec's chief medical officer. Another of Hingston's cohorts, Brannen had been the fastest skater of his day while still a student at Loyola College, and he was a member of the Montreal Shamrocks hockey team when it won the Stanley Cup in 1899 and 1900. Brannen graduated from McGill in 1900 and began his general practice in the United States. The First World War brought him back to Canada, where he enlisted in the Irish Rangers. When the war ended, he became a provincial medical health officer and the physician for the Montreal Royals Baseball Club. As was typically the case with doctors who had served in the military, his word was law, and subordinates didn't dare question him. It was left to Brannen to sort out the new, emerging realities. The hospital began to ration food supplies – tea, coffee, sugar, and canned vegetables. Even patients were issued ration books, and accounting forms had to be filled out and sent to Ottawa. To compound the problem, all wartime staff hiring was subject to review by the National Selective Service Bureau.

The hospital was busy, and with the opening of an airbase at nearby Cartierville, it became even busier. Three staff surgeons did the work of six, clinical work was curtailed, and Dr. Goodall's blood bank was forced to close due to lack of staff. The nuns cut back on their use of gauze, bandages, adhesives, and plaster, and they further tried to cut costs by buying drugs from McGill's pharmacopeia. Certainly, Brannen's most pressing responsibility was to deal with the hospital's increasingly precarious financial situation.

"Because of the war the government can conscript assistance, but hospitals are forbidden to acquire adequate staff," Brannen wrote to Hingston on September 26, 1942. "We must safeguard the little children and helpless infants confined to our care. The lack of help and the type of help we must accept, is resulting in great hardship, and even tragedy may ensue if something is not done at once...the injustice is obvious as children's lives as future citizens, and the lives of soldiers are important from every point of view. This is just the beginning of a very serious situation and portends neglect of, and possible loss of life." During the war, it was the student nurses who kept St. Mary's running – 18-year-olds just out of high school who put in 12- to 14-hour days, working for nothing, looking after 20 to 30 patients, with only one graduate nurse on the floor. "You had to be obedient, you couldn't open your mouth," recalled one nurse who was there at the time. "Young nurses who came in with any suggestions or came in with new procedures were ignored. There were no unions, no such things as human rights. You did what you were told, and you liked it."

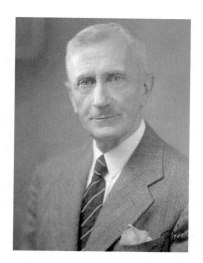

Dr. John Brannen, St. Mary's
first Superintendent.

Under the terms of the Quebec Public Charities Act, the province
was obliged to pay one-third of the cost of caring for indigent patients,
or $4 a day. But because of the war effort, St. Mary's was being reim-
bursed under the old rate of $1.62, losing more than $2 per patient
daily. "It is rather difficult to understand the apathetic attitude taken
by government which is not shouldering its just responsibility in
regard to caring for the sick poor. Simple arithmetic will indicate the
financial burden," Brannen complained. The cost of running the nursing school also escalated. Following Sister St. Simon's departure, in
1936, a series of nursing school superiors tried, and in quick succession failed, to balance the books. In spite of her many flaws, Mother
Morrissey had been right about one thing: a hospital and a school of
nursing needed to be treated as separate institutions, and it was folly
to shoehorn them into a single unit. Industrial management consultants Dufresne, McLagan and Associates were hired to target waste and
to recommend ways of increasing revenue. The consultants discovered
that the arrangement St. Mary's had with the Grey Nuns was financially inefficient. Four different departments were buying supplies for
the hospital. Observed Brannen: "The operation of the kitchen comes

under the supervision of the medical superintendent, yet the hiring of personnel is done by the sisters, and firing of personnel is the responsibility of the director of personnel." Because kitchen supplies were inadequately supervised, food from stores was being pilfered. As a result, the cost of providing meals varied day to day from "12.7 cents to 14.5 cents each."

The consultants recommended that a medical superintendent be hired to oversee a centralized system of purchasing. "It is now the practice for the funds to be handled by the Sister Superior in charge of nurses. We do not see any advantages accruing to the hospital from this practice, and we recommend that such funds and records be made part of the hospital's centralized accounting system." To implement the recommendations, the hospital would have to renegotiate its contract with the Grey Nuns, specifically article 2, which gave the nursing sisters authority to purchase all provisions, including food, linens, and bedding, as well as ordinary furnishings for the sick and generally for all the hospital staff.

Brannen met with nursing superior Sister Rose-Anne Rozon and asked the Grey Nuns to reopen the contract. On August 18, 1942, he wrote:

For some months the directors of St. Mary's have been greatly concerned over the financial and internal direction of the hospital. After giving a great deal of time and attention to the problems involved, after consulting with experts in financial administration, and upon their recommendation, the board is desirous of centralizing all of its authority for the financial operation of the hospital in a superintendent, who will be directed by and report to the board of directors. It is suggested that article 2, dealing with purchasing and the hiring and discharging of employees be deleted from your contract. Please be assured that this action is not in any way a reflection upon the efficiency and co-operation of the Reverend sisters. It is desired entirely in order that our board may function more effectively. It is absolutely necessary for us to centralize all departments if we are to curtail expenses and reduce our ever increasing deficit which has reached a very alarming proportion. A few years ago this deficit would not have worried us as we could count on the generosity of those who believed in St. Mary's to help us over any financial problems we may encounter. Today, due to high taxation and increased cost of living this means of balancing our budget no longer exists owing to war conditions, we cannot permit ourselves the luxury of a graceful and easy management, and we must cut all unnecessary expenditures, whether of a luxury class or otherwise, and in a great many cases, cut actual necessities.

It was precisely because of conditions during the war that the Grey Nuns were reluctant to reopen their contract. It hadn't been easy to recruit nuns willing to work in English. Training women to provide services in English to patients was an expensive proposition. "Under no conditions do [we]…feel any action [should] take place before we have a written document from the General Council of the Mother House," Rozon replied. The General Council met, and it concluded that bilingual nursing sisters were needed to replace nurses in its Western Canadian hospitals who had reported for active duty. Furthermore, if the Grey Nuns were to give up their control of purchasing, they expected some form of compensation. Bishop Gauthier was called upon to resolve the impasse, and he settled the issue by ruling that, "à cause de langue anglaise," the Grey Nuns would no longer staff St. Mary's. Their departure from the hospital during the war aggravated a growing list of administrative headaches, and the board remained "greatly worried" about the hospital's future – "whether it remains a private institution run as it was intended to be run, or whether it will be taken over by the government and operated as a private institution."

With the Grey Nuns gone, yet another women's auxiliary, the Union of Hospital Volunteers, with its own executive, was started, much to the consternation of the two existing women's volunteer groups. The

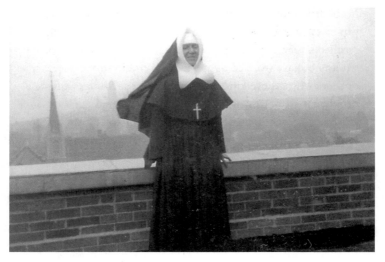

Mother Superior Mary Adalbert Rozmahel, seen here on the roof of the
hospital, brought the Sisters of Providence to St. Mary's in 1943.

new volunteers took it upon themselves to visit the public wards,
"bringing cigarettes for the men and home made candy for the women
as well as distributing magazines and scapular medals."

On June 1, 1943, 12 nuns from the Sisters of Charity of the House of
Providence in Heathfield, near Kingston, Ontario, agreed to replace
the Grey Nuns on the hospital's terms. The Sisters of Providence, also
known as the Sisters of Charity, were an offshoot of their French-
speaking counterparts in Quebec. The order was founded in 1861 by
Catherine McKinley, a dressmaker, who joined the community in
Montreal before moving to Kingston. Sister Mary Adalbert Rozmahel,
a quiet, determined perfectionist, was chosen to be the new administrative superior at St. Mary's, and Sister Mary Flavian Kearney would
take over as superintendent of nurses.

Rozmahel was born in Ord, Nebraska, but she grew up in Alberta.
Impressed by the way the Sisters of Providence had cared for her ailing
grandmother at the order's hospital in Daysland, Alberta, she decided

to become a nun. "Their charity to the sick could not be surpassed," she wrote. "No matter how difficult the patient was, they looked after them as if they were looking after Christ." Rozmahel was 20 when she joined the order, in 1913. She trained as a nurse in Brockville, Ontario, and she spent 17 years at that city's St. Vincent's Hospital before being posted to Montreal. In Montreal, she discovered just how difficult it was to run a hospital in wartime. The *Gazette* described the situation in an editorial: "To begin with there is a shortage of doctors, secondly there is a shortage of nurses because many graduate nurses have left to work in munitions plants, thirdly there is a shortage of interns. Young men who normally would have spent a year in a hospital are now going into [the] Royal Canadian Army Medical Corps directly upon graduation. Worst of all is the shortage of maintenance personnel. Orderlies, maids, cooks, waitresses are practically unobtainable and unless some are obtained soon, the hospitals will be in a bad situation."

Keeping staff was a problem, and the board complained about the increase in the number of untrained maids on the payroll. "There are too many of them holding up the walls," was a common complaint. The war brought with it changing mores and morals, and the staff became harder to discipline. There were chronic complaints of student nurses sunbathing on the roof, which they had nicknamed "the Tar Paper Riviera." One graduate nurse was expelled "for lack of decorum and shameful pilfering from a classmate." The story circulated of an amorous intern who would ride the dumb waiter to visit his girlfriend in her room on the sixth floor. One night, he pressed the wrong button and was delivered instead to the nuns' quarters on the seventh floor. There the embarrassed intern encountered an unflappable sister, who, without a word, shoved a tray of dirty dishes into his hands and pushed the button that would send him back to the kitchen.

CHAPTER FOUR

The provisions of mass sums of money for medical care is one thing; the way in which the money is to be used effectively, is quite another.
~ Reginald Percy Vivian

St. Mary's drifted into McGill's orbit in 1943, when the university, under pressure to increase the number of qualified physicians, extended its teaching season to 50 weeks. To be licensed in Quebec, a doctor needed four years of academic training and one year of on-the-job training. The university's acting dean of medicine, John R. Fraser, agreed to allow some of McGill's interns to complete their fifth year of on-the-job training at St. Mary's. A total of 12 interns from McGill were assigned to deliver babies, perform simple operations, assist in major surgery, and "take responsibility relative to individual patients." Of that number, four rotated through surgery, including a chief resident and a junior resident. As they grew in number, the interns required more living space, and they were housed, three to a room, on the fourth floor of the powerhouse, one floor above the laundry. Each room was equipped with a telephone, and when that phone rang during the night to summon an intern to a ward, all three would be jolted awake.

Then, in May 1944, the nurses were evicted from their temporary residence at 3835 Lacombe Avenue and moved onto the seventh floor of the West Wing of the already overcrowded hospital. Although the interns had their own bowling alley in the basement, there was no adequate space for more laboratories, clinics, or X-ray facilities. Built to house 200 patients, St. Mary's had become a 140-bed hospital. The task of organizing housing for nurses could no longer be postponed until the war was over. "The administration must face the responsibility of operating a training school for nurses by providing adequate housing and teaching facilities," board chairman James Kennedy insisted. The push to keep developing the hospital further and faster was symptomatic of chaotic wartime conditions. Donald Hingston, who had taken over as president of the Montreal City and District Savings Bank in 1942, was the ideal person to negotiate financing for a nurses' residence. He suggested "cheaper material and less elaborate construction than called for" and told the board that "more investigation will be required before any recommendation can be made."

Hingston did, however negotiate an $800,000 long-term agreement with the province's Liberal premier, Adélard Godbout, with the goal of putting St. Mary's on a sound financial footing. The government would guarantee the hospital an annuity of $40,000 for 20 years. "Hospitals have passed the stage where they should be considered only as charitable institutions," Hingston observed. "They are one of the largest businesses in the world dealing with the most precious commodity – health. They must therefore be run in as businesslike a manner as possible, but health cannot be sacrificed for financial standing."

Hingston was well aware that without government assistance, building a nurses' residence and expanding the hospital to 500 beds was too much to tackle all at once. Still, there was an urgent need to expand. After sitting through an exceptionally depressing meeting about the state of the hospital's finances, in May 1944, Hingston revived O'Donahoe's idea of getting the federal government involved in expansion plans. In a memo to the Montreal City Improvement League, he proposed that "instead of constructing a new building for returned service men who need medical care, the government take steps to enlarge St. Mary's and other hospitals in the city...If this plan was adopted, there would be great savings in the cost of construction of mechanical necessities: boilers, machinery, laundry equipment, electrical apparatus, etc. Such would reduce expenditure, increase speed of construction, give greater efficiency, and finally do much towards relieving under-hospitalization for the poor in different parts of the city."

Hingston also pointed out that while the new wings were being built, "existing laboratories and X-ray machines and the services of trained experts would be at the service of the officers of the government at little cost." Again, the proposal fell on deaf ears. In June, the Department of National Defence expropriated the Nazareth Institute – which had opened in 1932 a few blocks west of St. Mary's on Queen Mary Road – and renamed it the Queen Mary Veterans Hospital. Over the next 15 years, the government expanded the facility, which today houses the Institut universitaire de gériatrie de Montréal. Hingston was demoralized, and his health started to fail. "I haven't the strength to do much more pushing," he told Jack Dinan. "But if you still want to start the push [for hospital expansion], I will help you in every way I can. Get the young doctors on staff behind you and get started, and I will help you."

In June, Hingston retired as professor of clinical surgery at Hôtel-Dieu, and in July he stepped down as surgeon-in-chief at St. Mary's. Harold Dolan replaced him, Gordon Cassidy became chief of the Department of Medicine, and J.J. McGovern was named chairman of the medical board. "Time brings change to any institution," the *Canadian Register* commented when Hingston resigned. "Some of these changes are taken for granted, others attract attention and arouse discussion for a short period of time to be forgotten in the normal course of events. Of a different nature is the retirement of Dr. Donald Hingston....To stress the service which Dr. Hingston has rendered would be to gild the lily with a vengeance. His was the lion's share in the work, the sacrifices, the worry entailed in bringing a difficult and intricate undertaking to a successful issue."

Penicillin became available for civilian use in the summer of 1944, and the hospital ordered its full quota. Almost overnight, nurses went into overdrive to meet patients' demands for injections. A child guidance clinic opened as well, and it quickly grew as the war continued. The opening that year in Cartierville of the Canadair manufacturing plant for civil and military aircraft, and the subsequent development of the industrial corridor along Côte-de-Liesse Road, put an additional strain on the hospital's emergency services. It was becoming increasingly difficult to find qualified interns, and that summer a campaign to raise $50,000 for the nurses' residence failed. In June, the Allies invaded France; D-Day heralded the end of the war – peace was finally in sight. While plans for the nurses' residence were still indefinite and funds for it inadequate, the hospital's architect, Edward Turcotte, was asked "to proceed immediately" with blueprints for a three-storey residence, which would cost $420,000, "pending the acquisition of sufficient funds." Those plans were scrapped in August, when Premier Godbout's Liberal provincial government was unexpectedly defeated, and the new premier, Maurice Duplessis, ordered an immediate review of the terms and conditions of the $800,000 annuity ($40,000 for 20 years) that Godbout had promised to St. Mary's. At the same time, while the new government revised its healthcare commitments, it froze grants made under the Quebec Public Charities Act. In desperation, Hingston turned once again to Lieutenant Colonel William Patrick O'Brien and asked him to take charge of the hospital board. This time, O'Brien agreed. Hingston, however, would soon discover that his confidence in O'Brien's abilities was misplaced.

In June 1945, McGill again approached St. Mary's for help in establishing a teaching hospital "where young doctors could receive training and experience that would enable them to take their places in the foremost ranks of their profession." Many of the doctors who had gone to war had limited medical experience, and those who were being demobilized required refresher courses and postgraduate training. McGill had started offering "special courses to enlisted medical men of comparatively small experience," but it could not accommodate the demand.

While St. Mary's was not yet qualified to offer residents hands-on training, McGill wanted the hospital to provide other "professional services that are adjunct to the medical staff." As Stanley Brice Frost writes in his two-volume history *McGill University: For the Advancement of Learning*, "a crisis had developed in the education of medical students…wartime advances in medicine and the development of technologies applicable to a number of pathological conditions increased the knowledge required by the contemporary physician." McGill was falling further and further behind other Canadian institutions. Its residents needed to work harder than ever to keep abreast of what was happening. The door to increased cooperation between McGill and St. Mary's opened wider when Wesley Bourne, who had been associated with St. Mary's since 1924, became founding chairman of the Department of Anesthesia at McGill. Bourne disliked performing administrative duties, but because he needed to work, he had accepted an appointment as assistant professor, becoming one of the first assistant professors to head a McGill department. His work on respiratory, cardiac, hepatic, renal, and central nervous functions, as well as on electrolytes, hormone levels, hemogoblin, and hematocrit during anesthesia, formed the basis for the specialty of anesthesia. Bourne's assistant, Peter O'Shaunessey, replaced him as chief anesthetist at St. Mary's.

O'Shaunessey was born in Elmsdale, Nova Scotia, but, as the son of a mining engineer, he had grown up in Northern Ontario. A quiet, self-effacing workaholic, who all of his life shaved two years from his 1897 birthdate, O'Shaunessey was apprenticed to a doctor in Haileybury, Ontario. He then enrolled in medicine at McGill, and in 1922 he obtained his degree. According to Jack Dinan, who returned to St. Mary's from the war in 1945, O'Shaunessey was "the rock upon which the department grew and developed. I don't think anyone in my experience carried the name Peter with more justification." O'Shaunessey proved to be popular with the nurses too, offering them training that other doctors didn't. He assisted in Bourne's classes, and thus became the first doctor from St. Mary's to receive a McGill appointment exclusively on the basis of his work at St. Mary's. Bourne and O'Shaunessey started screening young McGill residents and sending them on to St. Mary's. Many of the doctors they dispatched had wider experience than the older general practitioners on staff. As the ranks of these residents at St. Mary's swelled, McGill's influence at the hospital became pervasive. More and more residents in surgery, medicine, and other specialties went from McGill to St. Mary's for training.

The immediate postwar period saw the end of the era of personalized medicine. The old approach was replaced by a more sophisticated understanding of medical techniques. It was a period of remarkable growth at St. Mary's. The medical board increased pressure on the hospital board to approve an addition to the hospital. "In recent years, and through an agreement with McGill University, our interns have come to us from the graduating class in medicine. Students required to name a hospital of their choice have shown an increasing preference for St. Mary's," read a memo from the medical board to hospital board chairman James Kennedy. "Unfortunately, the interns' quarters are also too small, and must be enlarged if the hospital is to expand its facilities. It is the unanimous opinion of the medical board that this can be accomplished by the construction of a hospital wing rather than by building a separate home for the nurses at the present time or in the near future."

In spite of the growth, or perhaps because of it, 1946 proved to be one of the hospital's most discouraging years in terms of finances. "The business of running St. Mary's is in trouble, and unless that business receives some financial injection, St. Mary's will be in serious danger," building committee chairman James Gallagher stated bluntly. "Hospitals are often compared to hotels, but they go much further. It is found two employees are needed for every patient as opposed to one for the hotel guest."

In February, Hingston went to Quebec City to plead for increased government support. Although the meeting with Premier Duplessis and his minister of health, Dr. Albiny Paquette, was cordial, nothing came of it. On February 14, Hingston wrote to Paquette asking him to exert whatever influence he had with Duplessis to get the premier to honour the previous government's commitment to St. Mary's. But Paquette had no influence other than that which Duplessis permitted him, and appeals for aid fell on deaf ears.

The board had already paid $25,000 for land to the east of the hospital on which it planned to erect the nurses' residence, but by August, "owing to the hospital's lack of sufficient funds," it decided against proceeding with construction. Fundraising had become a never-ending, tedious obligation, and there was a limit to the support St. Mary's could expect from its traditional base – the English-speaking Catholic community. Most donations to the hospital were now coming from Protestants, and from a surprising number of Jews. Beds remained at a premium, and the waiting list for admission had started to grow. Only the most urgent cases could be accommodated. "This has led to increased demands for both nursing care and diagnostic facilities," the board was told. "Housing conditions, particularly on the 7th floor, are deplorable, and such as gravely to endanger the health of the nurses. The laboratories and X-ray departments are of insufficient size and should be enlarged."

In October, the hospital increased the daily rates it charged patients: semi-private rooms went from $4.50 to $5.50; private rooms, from $6.50 to $8; and deluxe suites, from $8 to $10. In spite of the increases, St. Mary's remained chronically underfunded. Technologically, it was not keeping pace with other hospitals, and the strain was obvious. "Every day the list of our patients grows, and we can do absolutely nothing to help these unfortunate cases," Aloysius Chopin complained to provincial health minister Paquette. "Before the last election, we had a promise of $800,000, but that has been broken. We want you to come to the assistance of our patients and come to the assistance of our hospital. Children's lives as future citizens and soldiers are as important from every point of view. Why cannot the government still keep in its services men of the lower medical classifications, or why could they not assist us to bring the salaries of the employees we now have up to a living wage?"

St. Mary's was not the only hospital in financial straits. In his survey of medical facilities on the Island of Montreal, Reginald Percy Vivian, professor of health and social medicine at McGill, recognized a need "for all groups in the English-speaking community to combine their efforts in a co-ordinated manner so that the objective of better healthcare may be achieved." To avoid expensive duplication of services, Vivian recommended even stronger ties between St. Mary's and McGill University. In 1946, federal health minister Brooke Claxton earmarked monies for more hospitals, but jurisdictional barriers still had to be overcome. Healthcare remained a provincial jurisdiction, and until Quebec and Ontario signed tax agreements with Ottawa, the funds could not be dispersed. On November 22, 1946, Claxton, along with federal Minister of Defence Douglas Abbott and Mayor of Montreal Camillien Houde, attended the St. Mary's Ball at the Windsor Hotel as guests. That year, the Ladies Auxiliary and the Maternity Committee set their differences aside and worked together to make the evening a glittering social success. However, the truce between the two groups was short-lived – tensions were renewed because the junior maternity committee sold 600 of the 800 ball tickets, but the senior women's group gave it only $400 as its share of the proceeds.

In 1947, Patrick O'Brien became chairman of the hospital board. His son Flying Officer Henry James Stuart O'Brien had been killed in action in 1944, and in his memory, O'Brien and his wife endowed St. Mary's with a gift of 300 milligrams of radium. Another of O'Brien's sons, Colonel William Lawrence Stewart, had been seriously injured when his plane was shot down after a raid on the Ruhr Valley. He had served as aide-de-camp to Canada's Governor General, the Earl of Athlone, before joining his father on St. Mary's Board of Directors. His social connections weren't of much help. That year, the hospital lost $70,000, and plans to build the nurses' residence remained in limbo. "With the public givers being gradually drained of their surplus income, and with the gradual increases in hospital deficits, the day may not be far distant when government may be forced to take over hospitals, and that will be a sad day indeed, as one can well imagine how bureaucracy will serve the sick," Chopin again warned. "This hospital will either cease to exist, or be absorbed by some national health scheme which will be dictatorial and commandeer by law all the powers invested in hospital boards."

In spite of the hospital's financial difficulties, the board was able to report that staff morale was excellent. "A complete liaison between the department heads and the general operating members is so high that there is constant teaching and encouragement for individuals. The attending staff is a closely knit organization that has a good general attitude towards the institution; 50 percent of the staff are outstandingly interested in their work and have carried through. There are many M.D.s in the city who are anxious to have hospital privileges at St. Mary's who cannot be accepted because of lack of space to care for patients."

St. Mary's was doing well by paying scrupulous attention to basic patient care, by adhering to time-tested methods, and by conducting regular critiques of its overall performance. Its social standing in the community was elevated on November 7, 1947, when the first St. Mary's Ball under viceregal patronage was held at the Windsor Hotel. Taking as its theme the popular Bing Crosby movie *The Bells of St. Mary's*, the event was billed as "the Belles of St. Mary's." Canada's governor general, the newly minted British viscount Harold Alexander, 1st Earl Alexander of Tunis, who had commanded the Allied armies in Italy during the Second World War, was the honoured guest. The St. Mary's Hospital Maternity Committee, still piqued at being shortchanged by the Ladies Auxiliary at the previous year's ball, refused to sell tickets and boycotted the event; nevertheless, $6,000 was raised. But such social successes could not mask the hospital's serious financial situation. No amount of private fundraising could meet the hospital's requirements.

Throughout the war, the maternity unit at the hospital had been bursting at the seams. In 1946, Gerald Altimas was brought in to replace the retiring Dunstan Gray and to consolidate the departments of Obstetrics and Gynecology. Altimas was a railway conductor's son who had grown up in St-Henri and had worked as ship's steward to pay his way through Loyola College. A natural athlete, he was responsible for reviving Loyola's lacrosse team in the 1920s, and he went on to play hockey and football at McGill, where he studied medicine. Altimas obtained his license to practise in 1931 then interned at St. Mary's for a year before leaving Montreal to study obstetrics at Johns Hopkins. Tom Altimas recalls that his father had a voracious appetite for work and "considerable practical experience, more than he claimed on his CV. He was on staff at both the Catherine Booth and the Reddy Memorial, and he took on more maternity cases than he could handle. He was one of those people who just couldn't say no."

Altimas loved Tchaikovsky. In the operating suite, he would often play a recording of the First Piano Concerto with the volume cranked up. He was ambitious and had newfangled ideas about how the departments should be integrated, which made the superintendent of nurses, Sister Hildegarde, and the supervisor of the Obstetrics department, Sister Mercy, uneasy. The trend to biomedical science and technology had made the hospital's existing research facilities obsolete. Altimas moved quickly to ensure that St. Mary's kept pace with the latest innovations in obstetrics and gynecology, and, with Gray, he laid the foundations for what would become the hospital's greatest strength. During his first year in charge of the department, 1,458 babies were born – including the first set of triplets – with only one maternal death. In his third annual report on the department, Altimas was able to take credit for reducing the number of newborn deaths, "largely because of a more efficient use of the oxygen apparatus supplied to the nursery by the maternity committee." While conditions in the nursery had improved, Altimas was still concerned, because "with our present facilities, we have reached the limit of our capacity...there is still a crying need for public beds, both for the care of patients and for the training of interns."

After the war, Canadians increasingly regarded access to healthcare as a right, not a privilege. One public opinion poll indicated that in 1948, 73 percent of the population wanted more hospitals and free medical clinics. That year, St. Mary's handled 5,265 patients, and, "despite strictest measures and constant and close supervision of all expenditures," it saw its deficit increase by 76 percent to $129,000. "Voluntary hospitals are passing through the most critical period of

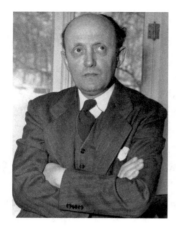

Dr. Karl Stern built St. Mary's
Department of Psychiatry.

their history and cannot continue their less-than-cost policy unless
federal and provincial governments recognize that modern hospital
care is increasingly expensive," cautioned Aloysius Chopin. "If the
present system breaks down – and it is dangerously near the breaking
point – then governments will learn first hand, and at heavy cost what
it is to care for the sick."

In an attempt to stimulate public support for its fundraising efforts,
St. Mary's sponsored its first open house – "Hospital Day" – on June 12,
which gave the public an opportunity to tour the hospital and at the
same time contribute to its support. Generally speaking, patients were
happy with the care they received at St. Mary's. The sentiment expressed most often in their letters of appreciation dating from the
1940s is that the hospital staff had shown them kindness. A typical
note came from a Jessie McLean: "The whole attitude of the people of
St. Mary's is one of Christian kindness. We received spiritual, physical
and mental comfort while we remained under its roof. Physicians,
surgeons, sisters and nurses were amazingly kind."

With the appointment of Karl Stern as first consulting psychiatrist
in the spring of 1948, St. Mary's began welcoming Europe's medical
refugees. Stern, a Bavarian Jew who had converted to Roman Catholicism, was an internationally acclaimed authority on menopausal

expression and senility. A quiet and reserved man, Stern had studied at the universities of Munich, Berlin, and Frankfurt before emigrating to London in 1938. There, Dr. Wilder Penfield had recruited him for the Allan Memorial Institute, which Penfield had opened in Montreal in 1944. Stern was on the staff of the Protestant Insane Asylum (which later became the Douglas Hospital) in the Montreal neighbourhood of Verdun when it became a McGill teaching hospital in 1946. In his autobiography, *The Pillar of Fire*, Stern described himself as someone "who had known the life of freedom, the perfect libertinism of European youth of the twenties and the hangover of nothingness and despair." This led him to search for meaning in Roman Catholicism. Eventually, in 1958, he would establish the Department of Psychiatry at St. Mary's. Later he taught at the University of Ottawa. His books *The Flight from Woman* and *Love and Success, and Other Essays* are still recommended reading.

Medical knowledge was increasing at a rapid rate, and many of the older doctors at St. Mary's were now out of touch. Stern was an exception. St. Mary's had outgrown its beginnings, but it was still clannish, and it was still being run as though it were a venerable Irish men's club. One doctor suggested that reciting the rosary each evening over the hospital's public address system would have therapeutic value, as it would reduce patients' blood pressure. The idea was seriously considered but never implemented. The hospital's special credentials committee lamented that cronyism was rampant and that only a few staff doctors submitted papers to recognized medical journals or attended medical conventions. Only 25 percent of the doctors, the committee noted, had even bothered to become members of the Medico-Chirurgical Society, and those who were accredited society members rarely attended meetings.

As chairman of staff meetings, Dr. Jack Lafave was the liaison between medical staff and the board, and he became one of the more forceful voices in favour of bringing in new blood and expanding the hospital. "There is a continuing waiting list of patients, which can only be partly relieved when the 6th floor is in service. Laboratories are

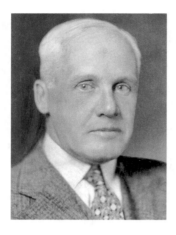

Board Chairman Patrick O'Brien
opposed hospital expansion.

over-taxed, and the X-ray department is growing and we need more accommodation for nurses and internes," he told building committee chairman James Gallagher. "A careful reading of our reports clearly indicates the need for immediate planning for expansion....Occupancy is being maintained at capacity, and at times exceeds bed complement, overcrowding the wards beyond the margins of safety."

Lafave distilled all the suggestions, reports, and resolutions from the general consensus, then presented them to the Board of Directors at a meeting held at the Mount Stephen Club in September 1948. Dr. Leo Mason was especially persuasive in making the case for a new wing – his presentation was remarkable for its clarity. The hospital had already floated bond issues to finance the nurses' residence, and Mason suggested that they finance a 400-room addition in the same way. Board chairman Patrick O'Brien told Mason that the doctors' proposal was little more than "wishful thinking." He insisted that the gap between what the doctors wanted and what the hospital could afford was extremely wide. O'Brien had never been a great fan of St. Mary's, and perhaps under the influence of one drink too many he unleashed his anger. What St. Mary's needed was not more beds, he exploded. It needed better doctors. Even if they got their new wing, the doctors on staff wouldn't know what to do with it, he raged, adding, "If there is no improvement shortly, there will be no promotions, and in some cases, present appointments will not be renewed."

Tempers flared on both sides, harsh words were exchanged, and O'Brien smashed a glass on the table, bringing the argument to an abrupt conclusion. "We had planned to start expansion by soliciting funds before the big McGill hospitals," Jack Dinan explained. "But this donnybrook set us back several years."

CHAPTER FIVE

There was no discrimination among the different nationalities, races or
religious denominations. St. Mary's was tolerant, accepting of everyone.
~ Dr. Karl Essig

In the first of a series of commemorative events to mark the 25th anniversary of the opening of the first St. Mary's in Shaughnessy House, Donald Hingston laid the cornerstone for the nurses' residence on January 25, 1949. As Bishop Lawrence Whelan blessed the stone, he declared that the new facility for 108 nurses would allow the hospital "to grow and provide even greater service to the community." Hingston wasn't so sure – if anything, he thought the expansion was short-sighted. "If the nurses home now being built will accommodate 108, we will necessarily have shortage of approximately 76 nurses," he complained to building committee chairman James Gallagher. "If it is not too late, please place another floor on the nurses home. This would accommodate another 25 to 32 nurses." Without the additional floor, he argued, "the efficiency of the hospital will suffer, and with it the hospital's good name." As well, Hingston didn't see any need for St. Mary's to hire graduates from other nursing schools to make up for the anticipated staff shortages. "These nurses do not know the ropes at St. Mary's," he wrote. "Graduate nurses pick and choose a bit. It is not always easy to get them for certain nasty cases nor for cases at unpleasant hours. Our nurses do what they are told. Many nice things are said about our nurses – they spend three years in training with us then spread around the country the principles and practices they have learned at St. Mary's. Why not increase that good work if we can? Surely the result justifies it."

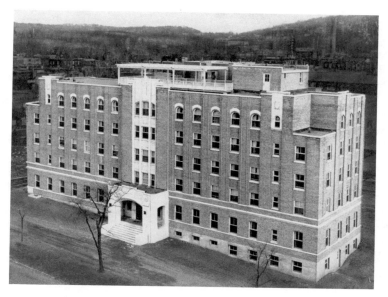

The nurses' residence, built in 1950, could accommodate
108 nursing students.

Hingston also cautioned against adding a wing to the back of the
hospital. "Let us proceed carefully," he wrote. "It is so easy for us to
meander along the wrong road, but above all let us get all the worthwhile information we can before deciding."

A campaign to raise $118,000, called "Keep the Door Open," was
launched in the spring and met its objective. The Silver Anniversary
Ball on November 4, with honoured guests Governor General Lord
Alexander of Tunis and Prime Minister Louis St. Laurent, was also a
success. The *Montreal Star* pronounced the evening "one of the most
brilliant gatherings in the history of St. Mary's." Three months later,
on February 2, 1950, Bishop Whelan blessed the new nurses' residence and told those assembled for the occasion that the federal
minister of health and welfare, Paul Martin Sr., had given the hospital $82,000 to add 82 more beds. "Duplessis raised a bit of a fuss and
claimed the grant usurped his role of deciding priorities in the

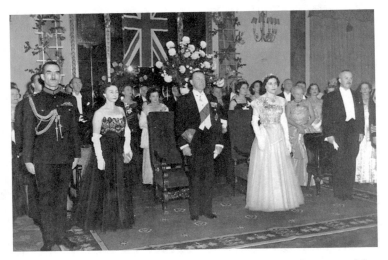

Governor General Lord Alexander and Lady Tunis, viceregal patrons of the hospital's 25th Anniversary Ball, November 4, 1949.

health field," Martin later recalled. "But the hospital ignored the Quebec premier's objections and took the money." Nursing school head Sister Mary Hildegarde reported that the new residence "marks a great advancement in the march of progress of our School of Nursing…we now have a residence carefully planned and adequately furnished." But, she added, "some form of direct connection between the residence and the hospital, such as a tunnel or an overhead, would seem to be a necessity."

To celebrate the residence opening, Hingston threw an oyster party for the interns three weeks later, an event that eventually morphed into the annual Hingston Dinner, a tradition to which St. Mary's adheres to this day. Hingston started to write a history of the hospital, cautioning the reader that his account "may seem egotistical. One must realize that I was always at the centre of the movement, and thus cannot escape a certain egotism." He never finished the work. His health deteriorated, and that summer he slipped into "helplessness and silence" for several weeks and then died on November 15, 1950. On his passing, the *Gazette* remarked, "Those who knew him as a surgeon have known that like his father before him, no man had learned better how to enter into the fears and anxieties of those he attended."

Hingston's death was but one of a number of changes that would affect the hospital. Sister Mary Adalbert Rozmahel had resigned as head of the nursing school and was replaced by Sister Hildegarde. Born Mary Ann Rushman in Crysler, Ontario, Sister Hildegarde grew up in Tupper Lake, New York. She took her vows in 1916, obtained her degree in music from the Royal Conservatory in Toronto, and for 20 years taught music at Providence Manor in Kingston. Her career as an administrator began at St. Mary's. When Sister Hildegarde, cheerful and indefatigable, assumed her duties, the Timmins family had just donated their Île Cadieux property on Lake of Two Mountains to serve as a summer home for the exclusive use of the sisters. That autumn, George Bartel was brought in from Minnesota to run the hospital. Bartel came to Montreal from Minneapolis, where he had been in charge of St. Barnabas Hospital. He had also been a Kewaunee County school superintendent and had served in the South Pacific during the war as a United States Navy commander. A graduate of the University of Chicago, Bartel had a master's degree in hospital administration; his thesis was entitled "Examining the Position of the Hospital."

After the war, St. Mary's began acquiring specialists of its own, among them Guy E. Joron, who had a special interest in metabolic diseases and toxicology. Joron also had an appointment at the Montreal General Hospital. A notary's son, Joron, like so many others on staff, had been schooled by Jesuits at Loyola College before obtaining his medical degree from McGill in 1941. He had served in the Royal Canadian Air Force during the Second World War and had been assigned to study Inuit people working in Newfoundland and northern Saskatchewan in order to better understand the effects of cold weather on troops and their equipment. After this, Joron was sent to Washington, D.C., to study tropical medicine. By war's end, he had completed three years of residency at the Montreal General Hospital followed by a year's fellowship at Nuffield College, Oxford, but he had gained little experience with patients. A model of concision, tactful yet decisive, Joron would later prove to be an excellent administrator, ideally suited to the job of fostering an academic atmosphere at the hospital. He was attracted to St. Mary's precisely because it was becoming more and more cosmopolitan.

Unlike other hospitals in the city, by the early 1950s, St. Mary's had attracted an odd mix of foreign-born doctors, nurses, and interns. "Young to middle aged, they were of a different medical maturity," noted one of the admired newcomers, Karl Essig, who had been a submarine officer in the German Navy. It seemed that medicine had been in the Essig family genes for several generations: Karl Essig's father was a doctor, his grandfather was a doctor, and his great-grandfather was one too. Essig obtained his medical degree from the University of Tübingen and was known as a doctor's doctor – first-rate, cool, and dispassionate. He left St. Mary's for a year during the building of the Distant Early Warning System (DEW) to serve as director of health services at a DEW construction site in Ungava. When he returned to the Department of Medicine, he worked in the health office caring for the medical staff. Later, he was named chief of the Department of Medicine. An astute diagnostician, Essig had an intuitive approach to patient care and a remarkable ability to glean important clinical information from those in his care.

Essig was but one of hundreds of European medical specialists who came to St. Mary's after the war to undertake their internships. It was mandatory for all the foreign doctors, no matter what their previous experience had been, to familiarize themselves with Canadian methods before they could be awarded a license to practise. Among these Europeans were: a professor of surgery from Sofia, Bulgaria; a Hungarian gastroenterologist, Jeno Solymar; another Hungarian expatriate, an aged surgeon who had practised in the countryside; an aspiring British anesthetist who had been a star rugby player; Gerda Liepina from Latvia, who had studied medicine in Innsbruck and completed her medical studies at the University of Kiel; Sophie Rygier, a pharmacist from Poland; guidance counsellor Constance Duhaime,

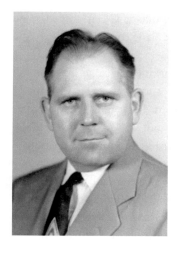

George Bartel, the hospital's
first administrator.

a graduate of the University of Leyden; radiologist Adolph Glay, a
Holocaust survivor and a very well-read man who had a great facility
with languages and who translated papers on radiology written in a
number of languages for the *Canadian Association of Radiologists
Journal*; S. Zuk, who came from Lubczyk in the Ukraine; and J.H.
Menetrez, who had fled German-occupied France in 1943 to join the
Resistance. But perhaps the most unconventional medical intern was
Bolívar de Peña, son-in-law of Raphael Leonidas Trujillo, dictator of
the Dominican Republic. Thanks to Trujillo's largesse, de Peña was
able to reside in a lavish Westmount mansion.

Pamela d'Abreu, a native of Georgetown, British Guinea (today
Guyana), became the first black person to graduate from the nursing
school, and George Matsumoto, the hospital's chef, was Japanese. No
hospital in the city was as ecumenical. The unique atmosphere was
featured in a 1951 *Montreal Star* story headlined, "Hospital Staff Like
a Little United Nations: Racial Boundaries Vanish at St. Mary's, where
staff members speak as many as five and six languages." However, in
an evocative essay entitled "To Be an Intern in the Early Fifties," Karl
Essig described the "enslaving conditions" aspiring doctors faced at St.
Mary's. "No union, no human rights activist, ever raised their voices

against the enslavement of young doctors that had been handed down by tradition," he wrote, tongue-in-cheek. Essig continued:

It was midnight when the interns' working day came to a close, and a late meal was offered in the hospital cafeteria. After the midnight snack, the interns' quarters beckoned. They were located on the 4th floor of the powerhouse, above the hospital's busy laundry room. Interns lived three to a room with Spartan furnishings. Unfortunately, there was only one telephone in each room, and it would ring during the night to call one of the interns to the wards, waking up the other two in the process. The intern on call had to get dressed and descend four flights of stairs to the tunnel, then rush towards the elevators of the main building. The elevators were not automated, but manned by two slightly demented identical twins who took turns and took equal pride in this important task....In the fifties the hospital maintained its own ambulance service and it was the law of the land that a medical person had to accompany every ambulance, not for any apparent medical reason, but to assist the ambulance driver manoeuvre the patient...into the ambulance, often a complicated procedure, especially in winter, when the patient had to be taken from the 3rd floor down icy spiral staircases so typical of the old houses. Because each ambulance trip was worth $5, it was a welcome addition to the intern's $50 monthly stipend. Having [experienced] the ravages of war, our generation was rather used to deprivation. Even though gas was to be had for 16 cents a gallon, no intern could afford to buy an automobile, no matter how old or decrepit.

A haven for foreign medical graduates, St. Mary's became increasingly popular as an ethnic community hospital. Yosh Taguchi, a Japanese-born Canadian who as a young boy during the Second World War had been interned as an enemy alien by the Canadian government, was a medical intern at St. Mary's. Today a leading urologist,

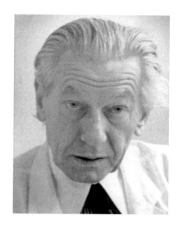

German naval officer Karl Essig was considered a doctor's doctor.

Taguchi recalls that because St. Mary's was a small hospital, he and his fellow young doctors were allowed to carry out procedures they would never have been permitted to undertake in larger teaching hospitals. McGill's principal, Frank Cyril James, took note of the evolving symbiotic relationship between the two institutions when, in 1951, he again wrote to the hospital board president, George Daly, to suggest affiliation. That year, Premier Maurice Duplessis had forced McGill to turn down a $615,000 direct federal government grant, and the university was seeking ways to maintain its flagging reputation. An affiliation with St. Mary's was in McGill's best interest. At the time, residency training was hospital-based, and the Royal Victoria and the Montreal General could not handle the growing flood of applicants alone. The hospital board of St. Mary's approved the amalgamation, in principle, "until mechanical difficulties that may seem necessary might be cleared up." Reaction to working with McGill was mixed. Some board members still harboured the unrealistic hope that Loyola, which was a liberal arts college affiliated with Université de Montréal, would be fully accredited as a university. If that happened, St. Mary's would become Loyola University Hospital.

Others at the hospital were concerned that if St. Mary's were to become too closely identified with McGill then it would be deprived of its own federal grants. There were also fears that McGill might run short of something and simply take it from St. Mary's – a hypothetical notion that was debated angrily and ad nauseum. The crucial issue was one of identity. It was obvious that in any proposed merger of the two institutions, the smaller of the two would have the most to lose. Some doctors on staff were afraid that affiliation would compromise the Roman Catholic identity and the autonomy of St. Mary's; others were concerned that they would lose their hospital privileges. The Royal College of Physicians and Surgeons of Canada, however, approved St. Mary's for graduate training, and both Université de Montréal and McGill recommended the hospital for postgraduate training in surgery. That led to an increase in the number of subspecialists at St. Mary's holding dual appointments with either the Royal Victoria or the Montreal General.

Harold Dolan had been a member of the medical board's administrative committee at St. Mary's since 1934; he wrote about the treatment of pancreatitis and spent as much time treating the poor as he did those who could afford his services. He was appointed assistant professor of surgery at McGill. Then, in February 1952, the board recorded its "keen interest" in McGill's offer of affiliation and struck a liaison committee headed by Guy Joron to examine the pros and cons. Soon after, Wesley Bourne, the eminent anesthetist who had been associated with St. Mary's from the beginning, began sending his residents to St. Mary's for training.

The 1950s were an uncomplicated, relatively stress-free period at the hospital. Everything seemed to be black and white, like television, which arrived early in the decade. It was a straight-arrow time of economic growth and medical advances, including the Salk polio vaccine. In this era, a bishop could, and did, piously declare that "There are only three kinds of people in the world: Communists, committed Christians and amiable non-entities." Mixed marriages, which meant marriages between Christians of different denominations, were a subject of lively discussion; almost half of all Canadians disapproved of them. Unwed mothers were ostracized, and in Quebec, priests rushed

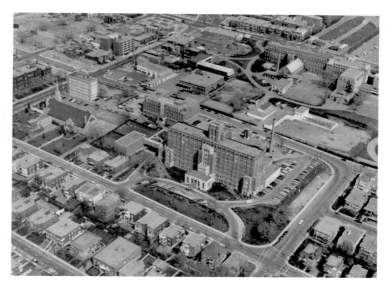

St. Mary's at the crossroads in the 1950s.

to baptize as Catholics babies who were branded "illegitimate" so that Protestants could not adopt them.

St. Mary's really came into its own as a hospital in the 1950s as the demography of the neighbourhood changed. The number of patients it treated mushroomed from 5,265 in 1950 to almost 7,000 by 1955. It was announced at one board meeting that "St. Mary's is at the crossroads of one of the city's biggest industrial developments, and has been called upon to handle a rapidly increasing load of accidents and other emergency cases of about 15 a day." At the same time, postwar inflation sent the cost of patient care soaring more than 40 percent in five years, from $7.86 per person after the war to $13.50 in the 1950s. "The road to a satisfactory level of public health is a hilly one," the *Montreal Star* commented. "No sooner is one rise surmounted than another is revealed just ahead. Not long ago, a major worry was the lack of sufficient accommodation…the concern now, is to finance the services which the expanded hospital system offers. The multiplicity of appeals for funds to cover deficits is proof enough that an acute situation exists, both acute and chronic."

In 1951, "in the interests of economy and better service to the public," St. Mary's joined forces with the Federation of Catholic Charities, and together they raised 93 percent of their joint objective of $563,000. But with only 178 beds, the hospital was struggling to stay afloat. Fundraising campaign chairman Louis Beaubien summed up the problem like this: "too much money going out and not nearly enough coming in. Not enough money is coming in because not many patients can afford to pay their bills. More money than ever is needed to improve and expand services and attract more doctors and nurses." In a further effort to make ends meet, the Ladies Auxiliary opened a coffee shop – just a small counter off the lobby – to raise money for a state-of-the-art sterilizer for baby formula. The women who ran the coffee shop, which sold hot beverages and homemade baked goods, kept meticulous accounts. During the first year of operation, they reported that 4,718 cups of coffee had been dispensed at seven cents a cup.

In October 1952, St. Mary's became the first hospital in the city to centralize its oxygen supply system, which allowed oxygen to be piped from a central distribution point to 142 outlets on the wards. That year, too, the federal government contributed $80,000 toward the cost of equipping a laboratory in recognition of Dr. Jack Dinan's "important results in cancer research, even though he had to work out of a basement." Dinan had discovered a relationship between serum copper levels and certain types of cancer. The money was used to convert the original ground-floor chapel into research laboratories. A new, 150-seat chapel and a rectory were built above the nursing sisters' annex and opened for worship on Easter Sunday, 1952.

Nursing shortages were on the mind of the federal health minister, Paul Martin Sr., when he spoke to the St. Mary's graduating class of nurses on May 8, 1952. There were, he observed, 400 fewer registered nurses in Canada that year than there had been in 1940. Martin suggested that St. Mary's hire more nursing assistants to "help conserve

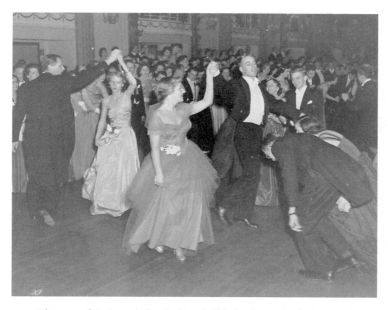

The annual St. Mary's fundraising ball helped sustain the hospital
during the lean years.

the limited supply of graduate nurses." He also reminded his audience
that opportunities for the hospital's first graduates had been "fairly
narrow, well defined and limited. Today, by comparison, all this is
changed. Nursing offers all kinds of interesting possibilities, specifically in industrial health programs, assignments in the far-flung
outposts of Canada's Indian Health Service, psychiatric nursing, teaching, supervision and civil defence programs."

Every department tried to keep abreast of the rapid advances in
medicine, and corporate donations were required to pay for the
special equipment this demanded. Measures to reduce the risks
involved in bringing babies into the world had been adopted a long
time previously, but if things did go wrong, St. Mary's was the place
to be. It had earned the enviable reputation of being one of the best

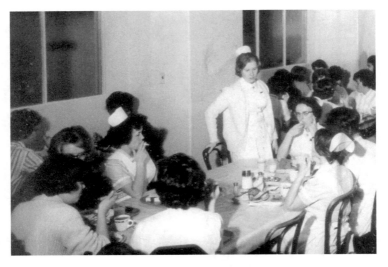

Even nurses smoked in the 1950s.

places to have your baby or to have your child treated. Still, even the best doctors can make mistakes if they are forced to work under stressful conditions. At least, George Mellen thought so. In the spring of 1952, Mellen suspected that his four-year-old son had been misdiagnosed at St. Mary's, and he asked to see the boy's case history. The hospital's directors refused, arguing that the medical records belonged to the hospital and, as such, they were confidential. Rebuffed, Mellen launched a $31,763 malpractice suit. When the case was heard, Judge Harry Batshaw ruled in Mellen's favour. "Hospital records are not privileged, particularly when it is the father of the patient himself who asks that it be exhibited to him for the purpose of making a copy," Batshaw reasoned. The decision set a precedent. St. Mary's has the dubious distinction of being the first hospital in Canada to be ordered by a court to make its medical records available to a patient. At St. Mary's, diagnostic errors have rarely been made due to inexperience or to technical factors, such as a mix-up in the laboratory. When mistakes are made it is usually because the doctor relies on pattern recognition, or diagnosing a disease based on the presence of a set of symptoms normally associated with that disease. Doctors who habitually use this method sometimes overlook the variables. Still, patient confidence in St. Mary's remained high. In the introduction to his collection of poems entitled *My Reflections on Hospital Life, Wise and Otherwise*, Donald Mac-Donald, a lawyer from Alexandria, Ontario, who had been treated at St. Mary's, offers these lines:

To those who need repairs my friend,
St. Mary's I can recommend.
The saws are sharp, the scalpels true
With steady hands to guide them through.
The nurses pleasing, skillful, kind
Are just the best that you can find.
The interns, serious erudite,
Watch over you both day and night.
And lest you should neglect your souls,
The sisters play their stellar roles.

The year 1952 marked another significant anniversary at St. Mary's. In July, the retired Helen Morrissey celebrated her 50 years as a nun. At the age of 91, she had clearly lost none of her spunk. Morrissey invited herself to St. Mary's, where she had the Auxiliary Bishop of Montreal, Joseph-Conrad Chaumont, celebrate the Mass marking her golden jubilee. During the reception afterward, Morrissey reminded anyone who would listen that she, and not Hingston (now deceased), was the "the true founder" of the hospital. Nine months later she was dead. In May 1953, Paul-Émile Léger, who had recently been elevated to cardinal, came to the hospital, resplendent in his scarlet robes, to bless the new chapel and to unveil a memorial plaque for Dr. Donald Hingston. The plaque is still there, on the left side of the main lobby, just past the bookshop. Mother Morrissey's name is nowhere to be found. To further honour Hingston, the Hingston Memorial Lectures were inaugurated; the first was given on October 13 at the Queen Mary Veterans Hospital by Frank Dixon, a surgeon at the Mayo Clinic.

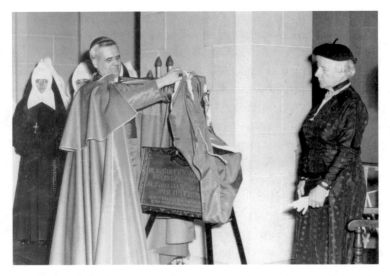

Cardinal Paul-Émile Leger unveils a memorial plaque to honour the hospital's founder, Donald Hingston, in the presence of Hingston's widow Lillian.

Starting on the day in 1947 when he took up his duties at St. Mary's,
Dr. Gerard Hurley, a chest surgeon from Cork, Ireland, had agitated
for a staff library. Hurley had trained in England, Switzerland, Germany, and the United States before coming to Canada in 1942 to be a
resident at the Montreal General. He would later perform one of the
first successful closed mitral commissurotomies (heart surgeries) in
Canada. Frustrated at the lack of library facilities, Hurley worked hard
to persuade the board to hire Lucile Lavigueur to start one, and he
finally succeeded. Lavigueur had a library science degree from Université de Montréal, and she agreed to take the job only because it was
convenient: she lived directly across the street from the hospital. She
set up shop in the boardroom in 1953, and whenever there was a board
meeting, the fledgling library had to close. Lavigueur didn't just build
a library. For the next 35 years, she remained in charge of the collection, and she was a resource as valuable as any of the books or
periodicals she stocked and diligently catalogued.

In 1954, the country's first hemophilia centre for adults with the bleeding disease opened at St. Mary's under the direction of blood specialist Dr. Cecil Harris. Harris had come to Canada from his native Scotland, where he had studied medicine at the University of Glasgow. In 1949, he arrived in Winnipeg, where he had been engaged to run a blood bank. Shortly after he took up his post at St. Mary's, the St. John Ambulance Brigade made him its provincial surgeon. One of the first patients Harris treated for hemophilia was Frank Schnabel, who, in 1963, would become founding president of the Canadian Hemophilia Society. Harris's expertise and his unorthodox approach to treating and supporting hemophiliacs was subsequently recognized by the society, which created an annual award in his name. On April 25 of that year, the hospital added a physiotherapy department that had a hydrotherapy room equipped with whirlpool baths.

The first major milestone on the road to integration with McGill University was reached at the end of 1954, when McGill's dean of medicine, Lyman Duff, an important figure in the history of Canadian pathology, helped St. Mary's to recruit an experienced pathologist who not only met the hospital's requirements but was also qualified to teach at the university. The Regina, Saskatchewan-born Dr. David Kahn was lecturing at Harvard and on staff at the Massachusetts General Hospital. Duff appealed to Kahn's "sense of patriotism," asking him to return to Canada and accept a dual appointment at St. Mary's and McGill. A hospital is only as good as its chief pathologist, and with Kahn's appointment, St. Mary's got one of the best on the continent. Kahn had obtained an arts degree from the University of Saskatchewan before enrolling in medicine at the University of Toronto. During the Second World War, he served overseas with the Royal Canadian Army Medical Corps. After the war, he returned to Saskatchewan, where he studied with renowned pathologist Norman McLetchie, a Scot whose groundbreaking discoveries related to using alloxan to produce diabetes in rabbits had attracted interest on both sides of the Atlantic. Bored with practising in small-town Wapella, Saskatchewan, Kahn moved to Boston to finish his residency at Beth

Israel Hospital; before going on to teach at Harvard, he worked with Benjamin Castleman, an outstanding human pathologist. Kahn brought to St. Mary's his organizational expertise and academic leadership. The first Jewish department head at St. Mary's, Kahn was "a medical man for all seasons," at the forefront of the movement to blend clinical medicine with medical science. His influence was felt at once. He was an intellectual who understood what was needed and how to obtain it. Kahn reorganized the hematology, biochemistry, and microbiology laboratories, and shortly after his arrival he became an assistant professor at McGill. Affable, gracious, and unassuming, Kahn was quickly accepted by the Catholics on staff because he was so competent and so ready to help. He mentored many of the doctors seeking fellowships, and, until his death in 2007, he was frequently asked for his advice on a wide variety of subjects, be they scientific, administrative, financial, or personal.

Another addition to the staff was Stanley Skoryna, a native of Warsaw who had studied medicine in Vienna. In 1947, when he was 26 years old, Skoryna came to Canada on an Edward W. Archibald Fellowship in experimental surgery from McGill. A surgeon and a scientist with wide-ranging interests, Skoryna had a number of theories he wished to prove, and he wasn't shy about lobbying for grants to finance his research. He came to St. Mary's with a reputation as a self-promoting cancer specialist, and in recognition of his determination, he would later be awarded the Royal College of Physicians and Surgeons of Canada Gold Medal for surgery. Skoryna thought that peptic ulcers were likely caused by bacteria, but he was unable to prove it. He also believed that smoking did not cause cancer. "Cancer is rarely produced in humans by external factors," he insisted, and he set out to show that the disease was the result of "an imbalance or lack of control by the various systems that make up the human body."

Karl Essig described the growing contingent of new arrivals as "an international conglomerate of medicine with a sprinkle of home-grown francophone talent, initiated into Anglo-American medical practice. There was no discrimination among the different nationalities,

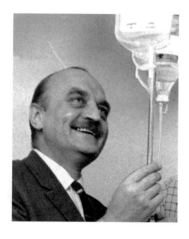

Dr. Cecil Harris opened Canada's first clinic for hemophiliacs.

races or religious denominations. St. Mary's was tolerant, accepting of everyone."

Around the same time, a couple of residents and an intern who would eventually help shake St. Mary's out of its complacency arrived: Richard "Dick" Moralejo, Benjamin "Ben" Thompson, and Constant "Connie" Nucci. Moralejo was 19 when he came to Montreal from Port of Spain, Trinidad, where his father was a doctor, to study medicine at McGill. After receiving his diploma in 1949, he did postgraduate surgery at St. Joseph's Hospital in Toronto, Queen Mary Veterans Hospital in Montreal, and St. Anne's Hospital in Ste-Anne-de-Bellevue before coming to St. Mary's in 1954 for his final year of training. Moralejo found swing music especially therapeutic. To relax, he joined a band and became its musical arranger.

Ben Thompson, from Savanna-la-Mar, Jamaica, had dreamed of becoming a doctor since he was 14 years old and one of his older sisters had died as the result of a simple appendectomy. Her death, combined with the illnesses of other family members and Jamaica's high incidence of venereal disease, motivated him to find a way to help the sick. He studied medicine at McGill and was awarded the Wood Gold Medal for excellence in clinical medicine. "St. Mary's gave the impression of being just a large family, a hospital for all people with

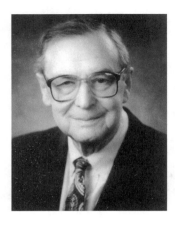

Dr. David Kahn, a medical man
for all seasons.

no regard to ethnicity or socioeconomic or other status," Thompson
recalled. "The fact that it was a Roman Catholic hospital was evident
only when the chaplain was called to administer the last rites. But min-
isters of other religious denominations also visited patients, so the
religious impact was not all that significant."

Connie Nucci, who came to the hospital as a rotating intern at
around the same time, was fluent in Italian, French, and English. An
accountant's son, he had completed an arts degree at McGill before
earning a degree in medicine from the University of Ottawa. In Ottawa,
Nucci had studied under Karl Stern, and, influenced by Stern, he had
toyed with the idea of becoming a psychiatrist before switching to obstetrics and gynecology. These three men belonged to the expanding
fraternity of Young Turks, all schooled at McGill, who represented the
changing of St. Mary's old guard of general practitioners.

The apogee of Montreal's 1954 social scene came in November,
when United States Senator John Fitzgerald Kennedy and his wife,
Jacqueline, were guests of honour at the St. Mary's Ball. Kennedy had
already staked out a position in support of Canada's decision to build
a seaway on the St. Lawrence River, with or without U.S. help. His
support for the project had been especially welcomed in Montreal.

95

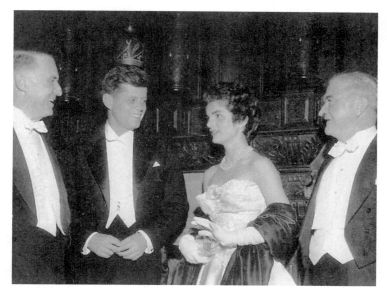

U.S. Senator John F. Kennedy and his wife Jacqueline at the
St. Mary's Ball, 1954.

However, no one at the time could have foreseen that within six years,
Kennedy would be president of the United States. The Kennedys had
travelled to Montreal as a favour to Edna Timmins, a St. Mary's
benefactor and a long-time Kennedy family friend – she had gone to
school with John Kennedy's mother, Rose. With his self-deprecating
wit and his natural curiosity about others, Kennedy captivated
everyone at the ball. And Jacqueline Kennedy was enchanting. Few
people were aware that one month before the ball, John Kennedy had
undergone a risky spinal operation, and it was by no means certain
that it had been a success. Leaving Montreal, he headed to a Kennedy
family home in Palm Beach, Florida, to convalesce. A convener of the
St. Mary's Ball, Genevieve Burke, learned of Kennedy's condition
after his departure, and she sent the senator a vial of holy water. Early

in January 1955, Burke received a three-page thank-you note from Jacqueline written on delicate eggshell-blue paper. The letter began, "I was so embarrassed [because it had been two months since the ball]. I hardly have the courage to write you this letter and thank you for being so thoughtful and kind." It ended with the line "I just hope it won't be too long before we can come back to Montreal where we had such an unforgettable time."

CHAPTER SIX

Faith in a hospital is born of experience; if patients are pleased with the care they receive, their faith in our hospital grows. Faith breeds confidence, and spreads, and spreads, and spreads.
~ Sister Melanie

Surgical teams in the 1950s at St. Mary's were often distracted during the summer by flies buzzing around the fourth-floor operating suite. There was no air conditioning, so windows had to be left open, and a nurse's aide was stationed with a bottle of ether to spray at insects that might slip through holes in the fly screens. Richard Moralejo recalls that once, while operating "on a patient of vast proportions," he was interrupted by a wisecracking colleague, Dr. Les Drake. A fly was circling the room. Everyone was preoccupied with the open cavity. Drake walked over to the table, looked deep into the gaping wound, and quipped: "You guys still looking for that fly?" As amusing as this anecdote might be, the fact that they still had to swat flies in the operating theatres was symptomatic of the hospital's growing obsolescence. So many new residents from developing subdivisions in nearby Town of Mount Royal and Côte-St-Luc flocked into the area that in 1954 a new municipal district had to be established. The superior of the nursing school, Sister Melanie, was concerned with the unprecedented rate of neighbourhood growth and its effect on the community hospital. St. Mary's, she warned, was becoming "dangerously overcrowded, with a 97 percent occupancy rate." Hospital facilities were stretched to the limit and the laboratories were too small to deal with the burgeoning number of patients.

To be effective, doctors and nurses require decent working conditions and the diagnostic tools that only well-equipped laboratories and state-of-the-art facilities can provide. Hospital management recognized the liabilities, and in the autumn of 1954, St. Mary's decided to embark on a 10-year expansion program – with or without government support. The ambitious $10-million program was designed to double the hospital's capacity. It called for two wings to be added to either side of the central tower on the eighth floor, a separate convent for the nuns (who would vacate the seventh floor), a chapel linked to the hospital by a skywalk, a wing behind the hospital, a new pavilion to the west of the existing building, a revamped front lobby, and additions to the nurses' residence. Stanley Clarke, a no-nonsense mechanical engineer who, beginning with a fleet of small ships on the north shore of the St. Lawrence River, had built a major transportation company with trucking and container-shipping divisions, was engaged to head the fundraising drive for the first phase of the project. Clarke was involved with the Federation of Catholic Charities and often quietly supported other capital campaigns in the diocese. He was not content to be merely a figurehead. With his engineering background, he took a major interest in the hospital's expansion plans. "He was very hands-on," said his son, Desmond. "He never shied away from rolling up his sleeves, raising the money, getting involved with the architects, and supervising construction. He was very detail-oriented."

Clarke assured the public that if St. Mary's reached its fundraising objective, then there would be no need for another public appeal for 10 years. The expansion plans were not based on future needs, he argued, but on current minimum requirements. "This appeal is directed to the whole community," the *Montreal Star* editorialized. "St. Mary's is a Catholic hospital, but its services are open to anyone who seeks them. Thus for every 15 English-speaking Roman Catholics who may be patients, there will be seven Protestants, five French-speaking Roman Catholics, and a number of Jews as well. Religious lines are not tightly drawn. The hospital is there to serve the community, and within the limits of its bed capacity and services, it has done this admirably."

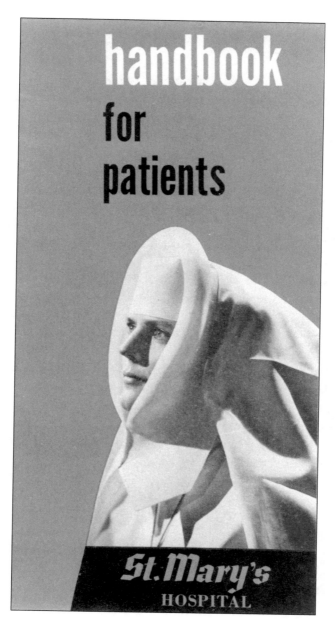

handbook
for
patients

St. Mary's
HOSPITAL

Sister Evelyn O'Grady was featured on the cover of the
manual governing hospital etiquette which was given
to patients in the 1950s.

In support of the campaign, the City of Montreal declared 1955 "the year of St. Mary's." Mayor Jean Drapeau offered words of encouragement, but city hall didn't chip in a penny. Drapeau was of the opinion that the city had done more than its share to get the hospital off the ground in 1930, and St. Mary's had proven that it could look after itself. "For a long time, while other hospitals were expanding, St. Mary's had made the best of the facilities it had by rearranging them, without asking anyone for money," Drapeau said, suggesting that St. Mary's could continue to get by. But St. Mary's had other friends in government – most notably, independent city councillor Frank Hanley, also the independent member of the Quebec legislature for St. Anne. Hanley had a knack for drumming up the necessary resources. If St. Mary's wasn't too particular about the source of the cash, then Hanley could always manage to deliver enough to help it through its small emergencies. The hospital could also count on the generosity of benefactors on staff, such as Dr. St. Clair Duffy, who, with his wife, Margaret, contributed $200,000 to the building fund. Duffy was a Prince Edward Islander who had studied medicine at St. Dunstan's University in P.E.I. and at McGill. He came to St. Mary's in 1928. Duffy dabbled in the stock market, and he did so well that he not only financed the renovations to the sixth floor of St. Mary's but he also endowed the Duffy Science Centre at the University of Prince Edward Island.

In the interests of presenting a united front to the public, Bishop Lawrence Whelan intervened to put an end to the chronic bickering between the Ladies Auxiliary and the Maternity Committee. In May, he ordered the two to merge into a single group: the Auxiliary of St. Mary's Hospital. Nadine Corbett was elected as the new auxiliary's first president, and it was left to her to come up with a new constitution. Kay Staines took over the direction of the increasingly lucrative coffee shop. Each weekday during the summer, a women's choir of volunteers known as the Belles of St. Mary's gave a noontime fundraising concert downtown, in Dominion Square (now Dorchester Square).

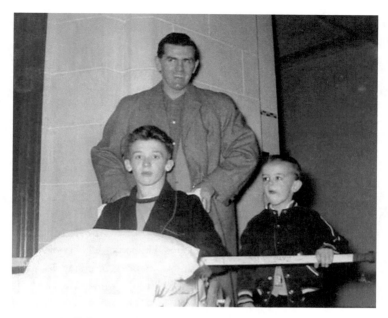

Maurice "The Rocket" Richard, with his son Normand (right), paid
a surprise visit to double-amputee Robert Vanden Abeele.

Thousands of people came and went through the doors of the
hospital that year. Among them was hockey star Maurice (Rocket)
Richard, who visited St. Mary's on November 1. Richard, forward for
the Montreal Canadiens, was still smarting from his notorious sus-
pension, which had sparked a riot at the Montreal Forum six months
earlier. He decided to drop by the hospital to visit Robert Vanden
Abeele, a 17-year-old boy who had lost both legs in a streetcar accident.
Vanden Abeele had written Richard a fan letter. Touched by the boy's
note, and with no ulterior motive, the National Hockey League's star
player arrived at St. Mary's unannounced to respond in person. When
it was suggested to him that his visit might be exploited to publicize
the fundraising campaign, Richard would have none of it. "There were
no reporters or news photographers present," maintained the nursing
school's mimeographed in-house newsletter, *Echoes*. "The atmosphere
was more of an uncle visiting a nephew." The following week, Richard
came back with one of his sons, Normand, to present Vanden Abeele

with an autographed hockey stick and the puck he had used to score his 429th career goal.

Aloysius Chopin, who had been with the hospital as a trusted accountant since day one, died in 1955. Shortly afterward, George Bartel left his position as executive director to become administrator of the Monmouth Hospital in Long Branch, New Jersey. Another American, Paul Meyer, was hired to replace him. Meyer's credentials were impeccable. A graduate of Brown and Duquesne universities, he had worked at hospitals in Brooklyn, New York; Clifton, New Jersey; and Bradford, Pennsylvania. He came to Montreal from the Instituto Clínica de Fisioterapia, Santa Rita, Cuba. Unlike Bartel, who was universally liked, Meyer had a swaggering sense of entitlement. To quote one of his subordinates, "He never quite fit in as one of the boys. He was much too fastidious."

By the time Meyer arrived to become the hospital's executive director, St. Mary's was treating more than 7,000 patients a year, occupancy had reached the saturation point, and, for the first time, patients were crowding the corridors. When he took over, there were 100 patients on the waiting list. One of the first things Meyer did was restrict admissions. His critics decried the move as a betrayal of the hospital's commitment to the community. Community had always been at the heart of St. Mary's self-definition. During "the year of St. Mary's," two teenaged schoolgirls, one from Villa Maria and one from St. Augustine, volunteered their services. Out of that gesture, a volunteer support group was born. Drawing upon four of the city's Catholic high schools, St. Mary's recruited 70 volunteers within six months. Christened "the Nightingales" by Hulda Lynch-Staunton, then director of volunteers, these girls carried meal trays, cranked up beds, and fluffed pillows, which allowed nurses, who were on call seven days a week, to take an occasional break.

Because St. Mary's was still regarded as being affiliated, "in a rather remote way," with McGill University, many of its younger specialists also had appointments at other hospitals. That had the advantage of improving specialized patient care while increasing the young doctors' experience and income. It also expanded teaching possibilities, which meant that an even larger number of house staff received accreditation.

Laboratory space was only granted by special request. Doctors such as George Vavruska, a dermatologist with a special interest in skin tumours who had come to Canada from Czechoslovakia in 1952, took advantage of every opportunity to use the lab facilities. Vavruska had studied with Frederic Mohs, a Wisconsin doctor who had developed a technique for colour-coding skin cancer tissue and who had created a mapping process to accurately identify the location of the remaining cancerous cells, which could then be removed with chemosurgery. Vavruska was the first to use the technique in Canada.

Following the Hungarian Revolution of 1956, Hungarian émigrés such as George Rona, who had studied medicine at Szeged and Budapest, came to Montreal. Rona wanted to pursue a career as an experimental pathologist and toxicologist. While learning to speak English and completing his North American pathology training at St. Mary's, he made the stunning discovery that infarct-like myocardial necrosis could be produced without cutting off the blood supply to the myocardium. When his training at St. Mary's was over, Rona accepted a post at the Lakeshore General Hospital and became a professor of pathology at McGill.

The language barrier was the most formidable obstacle for foreign arrivals. But, unlike the situation at other Montreal hospitals where English was the primary language, the situation at St. Mary's had evolved to the point that French was the common denominator. This was because so many of the new arrivals from Europe spoke some French. There was also a new breed of local trilingual doctors, such as Constant Nucci, who was fluent in Italian, English, and French.

On April 6, 1956, Bishop Lawrence Whelan turned the sod for a convent for the sisters to the east of the hospital, which would be linked by a skywalk to the main building. No one could foresee it, but for the next 15 years, St. Mary's would remain a construction site. To help finance the construction, the hospital sold a sliver of land on

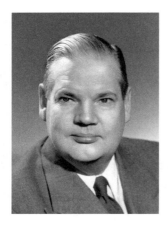

Dr. Louis Quinn was the driving force behind St. Mary's birthing centre.

Isabella Street. Later that year, a sub-department of ophthalmology opened under the direction of Gaston Duclos. A compact, dapper eye specialist from the Quebec village of St-Cyrille-de-Drummond, Duclos had graduated in medicine from Université Laval before serving with the Royal Canadian Army Medical Corps. After the war, he did postgraduate work in medicine at Harvard University and at the Massachusetts Eye and Ear Infirmary. He was also attached to the Queen Mary Veterans Hospital.

With the premature death at age 54 of Gerald Altimas in February 1957, Louis James Quinn, who had been a rotating intern at the hospital in the 1930s, became head of obstetrics and gynecology. Quinn had left St. Mary's during the war, in 1940, to serve overseas in the Royal Canadian Army Medical Corps. While in Europe, he had trained at the Chelsea Hospital for Women in London, and then he spent a year at the Sloan-Kettering Cancer Center in New York before returning to Montreal in 1947 to become an associate obstetrician at the Catherine Booth Hospital and a gynecologist at the Queen Mary Veterans Hospital. Like Altimas, Quinn had big ambitions for the department. He was determined to make St. Mary's the province's birthing centre. Described as a "rollicking, good-natured and talented surgeon who would not, or could not, take life too seriously," Quinn inherited a department with "a crying need for public beds," both for the care of patients and for the training of interns. "There have been no improvements…since the original construction of the hospital in 1934," he complained in the annual report. "Other Montreal hospitals allow husbands to remain with their wives during the first stages of labour. Because this modern trend is not permitted at St. Mary's, we are losing patients."

At an October 1957 meeting, the Board of Directors again agreed to explore the possibility of St. Mary's becoming a teaching hospital, and this time it instructed the medical board to "secure and maintain an affiliation with a university medical school." The board did not specify which university the hospital should approach, but it appeared open to affiliation with either McGill or Université de Montréal; it just wanted to ensure that the interests of St. Mary's were placed above any university requirements. This would be an important initiative: the board estimated that by becoming a teaching hospital, St. Mary's would see its annual budget augmented by 15 to 20 percent.

On November 10, the same day that he and Premier Maurice Duplessis opened the 800-bed children's hospital, Ste-Justine, on Côte-Ste-Catherine Road, Cardinal Léger also visited St. Mary's to bless the hospital's chapel, relocated to the third floor.

A number of unexpected staff changes in 1958 raised the bar for administrative and professional standards. Gordon Cassidy retired as chief of the Department of Medicine, and it was widely assumed that Neil Feeney, who had been on staff for 20 years, would succeed him. But Feeney had suffered a coronary thrombosis in 1949, and he had twice previously turned down the promotion. Instead, the Board of Directors looked to John Howlett, an associate professor at McGill. Howlett was a tall, jovial mountain of a man with an enormous capacity for work. He and his wife, Alphonsine Paré, were socially committed and deeply involved in Catholic action. (Alphonsine would receive the Order of Canada in 1980 for being a pioneer of social action.)

Howlett had come to Montreal from Newfoundland to study medicine at McGill, obtaining his degree in 1933. As department chief,

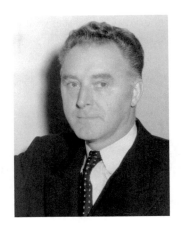

Dr. John Howlett opened the doors to affiliation with McGill University.

he remained on the McGill payroll and waived the $7,000 salary he was offered by St. Mary's, but he accepted a $1,000 annual expense account. Working together, Howlett and chief pathologist David Kahn forged even stronger links with McGill. Howlett reported directly to Lyman Duff, dean of McGill's Faculty of Medicine and chairman of the Department of Pathology at the Royal Victoria Hospital. This put Howlett in the privileged position of being able to assign a succession of senior residents and many McGill specialists to St. Mary's on a rotating basis. Among them were: Vincent Pateras, who arrived as an extern and would go on to become director of the Division of Nephrology; Antonio Guzman, a pediatric neurologist who later opened the electroencephalography laboratory; and doctors Ronald Stanford, David Stubington, and Frank D'Abadie, who would set up a coronary monitoring unit.

Harold Dolan stepped down as chief of surgery and was succeeded by Jack Dinan, who had been with the hospital since 1934. The fluently bilingual Dinan came from Quebec City, where his father had been the last English-speaking Irish city councillor. He had graduated from Bishop's University in 1928, then studied medicine at McGill. During the Second World War, he had served in Italy and Northern Europe with the Canadian Army. What most people noticed first about Dinan

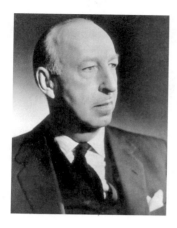

Surgeon Jack Dinan was the
hospital's historian.

was how big his hands were – in spite of their size, they served him
well during abdominal operations. At the same time, Guy Joron, who
had been quietly making his way up the administrative ladder, became
an associate physician in the Department of Medicine.

An audit that year revealed that Paul Meyer, the hospital's executive
director, had billed the hospital $14,000 for improvements to his house
in the neighbourhood of Hampstead. In May, Meyer was fired. In
search of a temporary replacement, the board turned to nursing superior Sister Melanie Coligan and asked her to pinch-hit until a new
executive director could be found.

Sister Melanie's temporary appointment as the hospital's executive
director began in 1958. Born in Morrisburg, Ontario, in 1912, Evelyn
Catherine Helen Coligan was one of 11 children. Her father, who was
on the local school board, supported her education, urging her to take
up typing, shorthand, and accounting. She was in grade 12 when
she decided to become a nurse and enrolled at St. Vincent de Paul
Hospital in Brockville, Ontario, for training. She had no intention of
becoming a nun. "Sitting in a chapel was never my greatest idea of
spirituality," she once said. "I was inclined to think that becoming a
nun was a rather strange and ridiculous step to take. My oldest sister,
Patricia, wanted to be a nun, and my mother was very much against

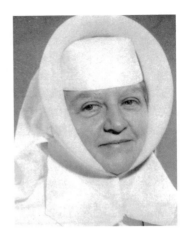

Sister Melanie. Her temporary
appointment lasted twenty years.

the idea." It was only after her mother died that Coligan decided that
the best way for her to serve the sick was to join a religious community.
"I didn't have that much to give up. Unless you had a lot of money, a
woman in those days didn't have a lot of professions to choose from,"
she recalled. "Lady doctors were not too well accepted; there were not
many lady lawyers, either."

She entered the Sisters of Providence order and made her profession of vows in 1934. As Sister Melanie, she was assigned to hospitals
in Moose Jaw, Saskatchewan, and Smiths Falls, Ontario, before obtaining a bachelor of arts in nursing education from the University of
Ottawa in 1943. She was then sent to teach science at St. Mary's, and
while she was on staff, she worked toward her master's degree from
Catholic University of America in Washington, D.C., which she completed in 1951. She went on to study hospital administration at the
University of Toronto, the Western University of London, Ontario
(which the University of Western Ontario was then called), and Université de Montréal, before being named nursing superior. Sister
Melanie was a practical, exacting woman. It was not hard to know
what she stood for and what she wouldn't stand for. As an administrator, nothing escaped her attention.

Once Sister Melanie was settled in her new job and confirmed as
executive director, her former position at the nursing school was

assumed by Sister Mary Felicitas Wekel, an equally formidable nun. Originally from Fife Lake, Saskatchewan, Sister Mary Felicitas entered the Sisters of Providence order in 1932. Like Sister Melanie, she had a master's degree in nursing from Catholic University of America. In 1967, she would become the first member of a religious order to be elected president of the Canadian Nurses Association. Sister Mary Felicitas set up a separate department within the hospital to look after the day-to-day nursing service. Also, she immediately set out to broaden the school's curriculum in order "to develop the highest ideals essential to a Christian nurse, to educate women in self-sacrifice and in the conscientious care of the sick, with an added appreciation and understanding of community health service." Working in tandem, the two sisters constituted an excellent management team, and Sister Melanie's "temporary" appointment lasted 20 years.

In November 1959, the hospital opened two five-storey additions to its south and west wings, which included an emergency admitting room. Interns were moved to the top floor of the powerhouse, and their old quarters were converted into an X-ray department with enhanced lab space. The imposing lobby, with its tiled floor, winding staircase, and coffered ceiling, was walled-in. A large basement auditorium was opened. Dr. H. Rocke Robertson had just arrived from Victoria, British Columbia, to serve as surgeon-in-chief at the Montreal General Hospital and professor in, and chairman, of the Department of Surgery at McGill University. As an indication of the growing cooperation between McGill and St. Mary's, Robertson inaugurated the auditorium with a Hingston lecture.

The first edition of *St. Mary's Medical Bulletin* appeared that fall. Richard Moralejo had launched the in-house publication to encourage doctors to write about their research projects, especially the "more unusual cases that are seen from time to time." Pat Madore, a meticulous, if somewhat reclusive doctor from Nova Scotia who specialized in thoracic surgery, edited the annual bulletin.

CHAPTER SEVEN

Socialized medicine might be free. But we should make sure free medicine doesn't mean defective medicine.
~ Aloysius Chopin

The first call for a system of universal healthcare in Canada was sounded in Saskatchewan in December 1959, when socialist premier Tommy Douglas introduced plans for an inexpensive, accessible provincial hospitalization scheme. This spawned a national epidemic of anxiety over the future of Canadian healthcare. The next decade was a period of turbulent change, and St. Mary's would be caught up in it. A thumbnail history lesson is in order. Douglas fought an election in Saskatchewan on the medicare issue on June 8, 1960, and he was returned to power with an increased majority. Two weeks later, on June 22, Jean Lesage and his Liberal Équipe de tonnerre (Thunder Team) were elected in Quebec, ushering in a decade of social upheaval often referred to as the Quiet Revolution.

In his first six months in office, Lesage rushed to establish his own Quebec hospital insurance program, effective January 1, 1961. The Quebec plan was by no means as far-reaching as that of Saskatchewan. Under the Quebec scheme, the government at last assumed the cost of patient care and established new per-bed rates for each day a patient spent in hospital. While the program alleviated some of its financial burden, St. Mary's was still responsible for its existing debt and for all of its capital and operating costs. The Quebec plan did not pay for diagnostic tests or drugs, nor did it fund research. Almost simultaneously, a federal Royal Commission was struck in response to continued demands from across Canada for a national healthcare program. Emmett Hall, a justice of the Supreme Court of Canada, was mandated to determine the best response to a situation that Canada's Progressive Conservative prime minister, John Diefenbaker, had described as "state medicine lurking around the corner." Hall eventually concluded that what Canada needed was a comprehensive national medicare program exactly like Saskatchewan's. The Canadian constitution clearly designates healthcare as a provincial jurisdiction, and the two largest provinces, Quebec and Ontario, didn't want any part of Hall's recommendations. Neither did private insurance companies or the organizations that claimed to speak for the country's doctors. Other factors that would have long-term effects at St. Mary's were also at play. For instance, all of this coincided with a Vatican Council that had met in Rome to promote a policy of more worldly inclusiveness for the Roman Catholic Church, which would involve transforming many of its institutions, including schools and hospitals. Within this uncertain context, St. Mary's struggled on.

As early as February 1960, hospital board president John Pennefather, a Montreal financier, was expressing alarm at the hospital's chronic $1.2 million accumulated deficit. In a letter to the province's deputy minister of health, Dr. Jean Grégoire, he stated: "The annual deficits have now reached a total far beyond what can be covered by volunteer contributions from the public....Most of our financial problem arises from the need to treat Montreal residents who claim inability to pay....Construction and modernization has been proceeding according to plan, but the stage has now been reached where the remaining building funds are insufficient to complete construction, provide furnishings and equipment. The hospital is now at a point where it must either obtain additional capital funds, or stop now, short of its goal, and continue to operate in its present partially completed form." St. Mary's, he added, was able to operate on a day-to-day basis "only by reason of two factors: One, a substantial bank overdraft....Two, the hospital is in effect using, as working capital, funds which are long overdue to its suppliers. This is a position which cannot be sustained much longer, and compounds the problem because it prevents purchasing material to the best advantage."

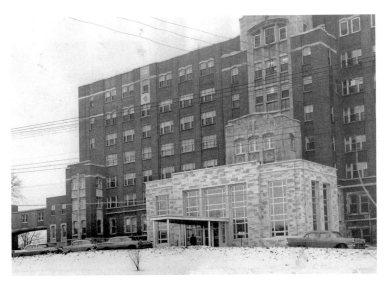

A new front entrance added in 1959 changed the hospital's façade.

St. Mary's had received a $40,000 federal grant to upgrade its X-ray equipment and another $177,000 to add a new front entrance, a lobby, a waiting room, and an eighth floor, and to expand the powerhouse. But by 1960, Montreal had 124 charities soliciting annual donations, and it was increasingly difficult to get people to subscribe to a hospital fundraising campaign. In any case, no amount of private fundraising could counter the steadily increasing costs of running the hospital. Furthermore, the old Roman Catholic parishes, which at one time could be relied upon for substantial contributions, were not as proprietary about St. Mary's as they once were. In a decision that, in retrospect, appears not to have been well considered, the hospital sold its tennis courts, which were located on property east of the nurses' residence, for a mere $81,334.50 to help finance construction of the new wing. The buyers, a consortium of St. Mary's doctors led by Moses Siminovitch, the hospital's cheerful chief of urology, built a medical centre on the site, which today is adjacent to the Côte-des-Neiges metro station.

The *St. Mary's Hospital Quarterly*, a glossy four-page bulletin, was launched in the spring of 1963 to raise public awareness of the hospital's financial predicament. This effort eventually raised $400,000. Corporate and private benefactors were recognized on May 1, 1961, when a stainless steel plaque dedicated "to the many people whose generosity has made this situation possible" was installed in the lobby. In unveiling the plaque, Bishop Whelan said that the gesture recognized "the outstanding Christian charity shown to the hospital by many industries and by thousands of people through monetary donations, as well as those individuals who have given their time freely as volunteers and as members of the Auxiliary."

The graduation exercises of the nursing school, held on May 19, coincided with the centennial of the founding of the Sisters of Providence. Mother Mary Lenore, the order's assistant general, delivered the convocation address to the 61 graduates in the auditorium at Université de Montréal. "Patients must never become mere numbers or filing cards," she reminded the class. "Efficiency is important and rightly expected of graduate nurses, but it must not become a cold, impersonal thing." Two foreign nursing students, Madeline Tcheng from Hong Kong and Annette Francis from Bermuda, took top honours in general proficiency that year.

"Medicare" remained the catchphrase of the day. Saskatchewan's initiative set off a firestorm of controversy throughout Canada after the Saskatchewan Medical Care Insurance Bill received royal assent in November 1961. Saskatchewan doctors refused to cooperate and threatened to strike and shut down all medical services. In Quebec, the Commission générale des hôpitaux catholiques de la province de Québec, which represented 80 percent of all the province's hospitals, including St. Mary's, complained about creeping government bureaucracy in the Quebec insurance scheme, about costs exceeding estimates, and about the seemingly arbitrary budget allocations for individual hospitals. Faced with encroaching government regulations, St. Mary's began to lose direct control over salaries and much of its budget. On February 14, 1962, snipping the ribbon to open the hospital's newly renovated seventh floor and inspecting the hemodialysis unit, Cardinal Léger sidestepped the issue. "In the present social climate, we have to be careful in making statements dealing with hospital problems," he told reporters. "We have to respect the law and see what will come out of today's decisions and actions."

Three days later, the hospital's board of directors met with Premier Jean Lesage to ask for $5.3 million in government money to continue its building expansion program. Facilities were becoming increasingly cramped, and, the board argued, if St. Mary's was to become a fully integrated hospital, then the hospital had to grow. Lesage was noncommittal. He told board president Leonard Hynes that the government would treat the request for capital funds and the hospital's accumulated debt as separate issues. It wasn't until Eric Kierans became Quebec's minister of health, in 1963, that St. Mary's found a sympathetic ear. Irish to the core, Kierans tenaciously supported the effort to secure government funding for St. Mary's. To ensure that the hospital was conforming to the new regulations established by the Quebec College of Physicians and Surgeons, St. Mary's named as its first medical director Jules Mercier, a Quebec City doctor who had worked at the Queen Mary Veterans Hospital. However, Mercier died three months after being appointed, and the post remained vacant for three years.

Vincent Pateras, who had gone to receive training in medical renal diseases at the George Washington University Hospital in Washington, D.C., returned to St. Mary's as an attending physician in 1963 and created the renal dialysis unit; the unit would treat patients with kidney failure from the Queen Mary Veterans Hospital and the Jewish General Hospital, as well as St. Mary's.

Under the patronage of Governor General Georges Vanier and his wife, Pauline, the annual St. Mary's Ball raised $10,000 for the building fund. Renovations to the West Wing began in the spring of 1964.

Every square inch of the wing was to be remodelled, and it would house a new kitchen, cafeteria, and dining room. The ongoing construction and the din of jackhammers were a constant disruption for interns and nurses on their rounds. "The volume of work performed in each department taxed the services to the utmost and in several of these services the load reached dangerously high peaks," Sister Melanie wrote in the 1965 annual report. The occupancy rate was at "a record and dangerous high of over 97 percent." The laboratories and the Department of Radiology were swamped with the growing number of patients, and facilities were under great strain. The number of outpatients reached a record 47,000; many of them were taking advantage of the Quebec insurance plan for the first time.

A nursing orderly training program was started to prepare new staff members to take up the slack, but, as Sister Melanie remarked, it was still the student nurses and the unpaid volunteers who made the difference. "We can never adequately express our thanks to the schoolgirls who arrive every afternoon, who bring a special aura of youth and well-being, the business girls who find time after a full day's work to cheer patients in the evening, and all the others who are here throughout the day manning the gift and coffee shops, bringing the gift cart to the patients, amusing the lonely children and helping in a host of other ways."

In the 1965 federal election, Lester Pearson's minority Liberal government, looking for a majority, campaigned on a promise to introduce national medicare. Pearson failed to win his majority. In order to survive in office, his Liberals needed the support of the New Democratic Party, and to ensure that support, Pearson had to make good on his promise. In spite of the constitutional hurdles involved, Ottawa came up with a scheme that would pay half the average national per capita cost of any provincial scheme. Pearson did not legislate the details of the cost-sharing programs (that would have been unconstitutional) but simply defined the federal government's notion of universal medicare. The provinces were left to design their own systems; and, as long as those systems fit into the overall grand scheme,

Ottawa would share the cost. Any provincial government that opted out would, in effect, have to explain to its electorate why it wasn't taking advantage of the plan.

The 1960s brought significant change to St. Mary's. It was a time of unprecedented social activism. Everywhere, authority was being challenged. Radicals of all kinds were contributing to the unsettled countercultural mood that was sweeping the country. Religion was now relegated to a secondary role. As a new, secular philosophy took root, Quebecers were being urged "to throw away the crutch of Christian schools, hospitals, social clubs and official Christian ideologies." The Roman Catholic Church withdrew from the business of healthcare, and St. Mary's was instructed "to put its religion in parentheses." Nuns shed their black veils and habits, and the nursing sisters became almost indistinguishable from the registered nurses. Charles Cahill, who had been the hospital's resident chaplain since 1955, left at the end of October, and Darrell Walsh replaced him. Walsh would be the last priest to have an apartment in the hospital. Walsh doubled as a handyman and was as eager to do repairs around the place as he was to look after the spiritual needs of patients.

As the government began to chip away at the hospital board's authority to determine hospital standards and set operating costs, the medical board took on more responsibility for harmonizing the professional and scientific requirements of St. Mary's. The hospital's doctors discovered that they could begin setting priorities of their own. Dr. Stanley Skoryna, who was director of McGill's gastrointestinal research laboratory, organized and led a medical expedition to Easter Island sponsored by the World Health Organization and the Medical Research Council of Canada. The expedition garnered widespread international acclaim, and Skoryna was honoured by the Chilean government. David Kahn was cited for his research into beer drinker's cardiomyopathy after he and another St. Mary's colleague, Dr. George Rona, discovered that the cobalt salt used by some Quebec breweries to give their brew an attractive foam head was poisoning beer drinkers. For a number of years, Kahn served as a consultant in bone and joint pathology for the Canadian Tumour Reference Centre, and he coauthored a number of papers with Rocke Robertson, by then McGill University's principal and vice chancellor. Cecil Harris went to Germany and Australia to chair top-flight symposiums on hemophilia. Another clinical researcher, Soichi Isomura, was working on developing a gas-exchange system that would extract oxygen from water, which could then be used to support life in underwater chambers. While all of this was happening, François Somlo came to St. Mary's from the virology department at Université de Montréal to open one of the first diagnostic virology laboratories in a Canadian hospital. Somlo specialized in obstetrical infections, and he introduced prenatal virology screening. He remained an active member of the St. Mary's community well into his eighties. He died in 1995.

In January 1966, the province's Catholic hospital association and its nondenominational hospital association merged to become Association des hôpitaux du Québec. French was introduced as the working language in hospitals, although the government still accepted submissions in English. St. Mary's was certified as an associate McGill University hospital for postgraduate training, and that meant McGill would take a much more direct role at the hospital in the teaching of postgraduate doctors. "Joining with McGill does not materially change the teaching carried out at present in the hospital," the staff was assured. "However, it will give the hospital a chance to expand to the fullest the postgraduate training programs." With that, the academic environment at the hospital was further stimulated.

But government bureaucracy has a logic of its own. Quebec's Department of Health wasn't prepared to finance McGill's teaching programs at St. Mary's, claiming that the Department of Education was responsible for all expenses incurred in the training of doctors and nurses. The Department of Education insisted that medical training came under the jurisdiction of the Minister of Social Affairs. Until the buck passing ended, St. Mary's was forced to dip into its special-purpose fund to pay the full cost of McGill's teaching programs, which came to about $100,000 a year. The situation was brought to the attention of McGill's acting dean of medicine, Patrick Cronin, but Cronin nonchalantly remarked, "If St. Mary's thought affiliation is going to get the hospital money, it's not. It's going to cost St. Mary's money." Initially, there was an uneasy feeling that McGill took it for granted that what was good for the university was automatically good for St. Mary's, and that the university's educational and scientific requirements took precedence over the hospital's day-to-day medical responsibilities. Sub-departments were being established at an accelerated rate, and again St. Mary's was running out of space to house them.

Again the hospital needed to grow. Following a meeting with Eric Kierans in February, the government gave the green light for a new 200-bed addition on the understanding that construction would "not begin before the middle of 1967." Kierans promised that the necessary funding would be approved at the first Cabinet meeting after the government's re-election. Architect Edward J. Turcotte drew up plans for "a seven-level wing" on Legaré Street. In March 1966, a campaign to raise $4.5 million was launched. Then, to everyone's astonishment, the Liberal government of Jean Lesage lost the June election to Daniel Johnson and his Union nationale. Tenders for the new building were called in October without any assurance that the incoming government, with its own ideas about healthcare, would honour Kierans's commitment. "Notwithstanding the results [of the election,] the Medical Board wishes to reaffirm its enthusiastic support for the construction of the new west wing," Jack Dinan told Stanley Clarke, who had become hospital board president in 1964. "The general feeling is that [such a project] is much easier to keep going than to start it up again should we let it stop now." Then, in November, Premier Johnson appointed a Quebec City technocrat, Claude Castonguay, to launch a full-scale review of the "ownership, Management [sic] and organization of hospitals." Not long after this, Quebec's new minister of health, Jean-Paul Cloutier, and the minister of state, Roch Boivin, toured St. Mary's and gave tacit approval to a hospital addition.

Accordingly, housekeeping moved to the West Wing of the basement and what had been the coffee shop became the gastroenterology and virology laboratories. The Department of Cardiology acquired a phonocardiograph, a state-of-the-art device for detecting heart murmurs. The introduction in the 1960s of mood-stabilizing drugs such as lithium, used to control mania and treat mental illness, caused a dramatic increase in the number of psychiatric patients being treated at St. Mary's. To accommodate them, the nuns moved out of the Sister House into smaller quarters in the nurses' residence, and the cloistered space in the convent was converted into a temporary ward for psychiatric cases. Nurses displaced by the new arrangement were housed in apartments within walking distance of the hospital.

As the hospital staff grew, the board recognized that doctors with substantial administrative responsibilities could no longer be expected to work for nothing. In 1945, there were 38 doctors on staff; by 1965, there were more than 200. From the time St. Mary's opened, department heads had not been on the hospital payroll – they volunteered their services. Like most doctors of the era, they depended almost exclusively on their patients for their income. That changed when David Power, a graduate of the National University of Ireland, accepted an appointment as chief of anesthesiology in 1966. Power was paid $7,000 a year "in consideration of the considerable amount of administration work that was required." When David Kahn was appointed to the hospital's management team shortly afterward, he, too, was put on salary. Because Kahn was Jewish, the hospital charter had to be amended by an act of the Quebec legislature to permit the election of "a maximum number of four people who do not profess the Roman Catholic Religion to the eighteen member board of directors." The act was changed on January 30, 1967, and at the same time, the corporate name of the hospital was changed from St. Mary's Memorial Hospital to St. Mary's Hospital.

As Canada celebrated its centennial in 1967, the ongoing debate over the future of medicare in Quebec sank into political quicksand.

At issue were doctors' salaries. How much should they be paid? A quiet tension took root at St. Mary's. Some specialists had grave doubts about medicare; general practitioners generally welcomed it. At McGill, the dean of medicine, Lloyd G. Stevenson, quit over the issue, and elsewhere residents and interns went on strike to ratchet up pressure on the government. "The day is gone when hospitals can exist on under-paid staff, over-disciplined nurses, and ill-paid and overworked residents and interns," reasoned the *Montreal Star*. For the first time in its history, St. Mary's was treating more than 10,000 patients each year, and the average bed occupancy rate was at 90 percent – "dangerously high in the medical and surgical services," Sister Melanie again warned.

In order to comply with revisions to the Quebec Hospital Act, the medical board was enlarged to 16 members "to harmonize professional and scientific interests, and ensure the highest standard of patient care." Olivier Leroux, an urbane physician with a wealth of international experience, was appointed medical director. A graduate of Université de Montréal, Leroux had distinguished himself by establishing hospitals in India, Jamaica, and Burma, and he had coordinated the youth division of the World Health Organization in Geneva. Louis James Quinn was named first chair of the expanded Medical Board of the Council. His wife, Maureen, pledged to raise $250,000 for the hospital's capital campaign, and she was elected head of the Ladies Auxiliary. That spring, Guy Joron was asked to become chief of the Department of Medicine, "subject to confirmation in writing that arrangements can be made with the Royal Victoria and/ or the Montreal General for the rotation of interns."

After Lloyd Stevenson's 1963 resignation as dean of the Faculty of Medicine, Joron had been given a part-time appointment as assistant dean. His most important duty was to serve as McGill's representative on the board of the Quebec College of Physicians and Surgeons. In 1967, when Maurice McGregor was appointed dean, Joron was offered a key position at St. Mary's: physician-in-chief. Joron attributed his selection to his being "the right man in the right place at the right

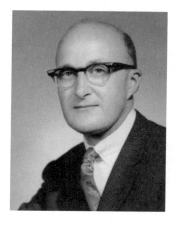

Dr. Guy Joron. The right man in the
right place at the right time.

time," ideally positioned to coordinate training and to facilitate the
hospital's amalgamation with McGill University. The challenge, as he
saw it, was "to insist that St. Mary's remain a Community hospital, to
continue to do what we do, but at the same time be important to the
research work of the university." But in April, on the day that Expo 67
opened in Montreal, Joron fractured his hip at the world's fair site.
His appointment was postponed for almost eight months, until he
recovered. William Bennett, the high-profile president of the Iron Ore
Company of Canada, assumed the chairmanship of the hospital
board, which was now known as the "Center Board." Bennett had been
president of Atomic Energy of Canada and had once been private secretary to one of the country's most formidable businessmen and
politicians: Clarence Decatur Howe.

The administrative changes at the hospital created a spirit of cohe-
sion. A temporary inpatient psychiatric unit was opened in July on
the seventh floor in the area vacated by the religious community.
St. Mary's was not immune to the galvanizing effect of Expo 67 and to
the heady "summer of love" atmosphere that was pervading the larger
society. During the fair, a Russian delegation led by Boris Danilov, the
Soviet deputy minister of health, and Dr. Anatol Saveczenko of the
Moscow Medical Institute, toured the hospital. Despite the havoc

caused by the ongoing construction, the Soviet doctors were impressed and commented on "the high level of patient care being delivered under challenging circumstances."

The summer of Expo 67 also marked the arrival at St. Mary's of Dr. Marvin Kwitko, one of the country's most creative and enterprising eye surgeons. Gaston Duclos recruited Kwitko for the St. Mary's ophthalmology department from Montreal's Hôpital Bellechasse. Kwitko was born in New York City, but he grew up in Brantford, Ontario, and obtained his medical degree from the University of Western Ontario in 1956; he went on to earn a master's degree in pharmacology from that university in 1958. This soft-spoken, methodical doctor had gained much of his experience at the Washington Hospital Center, a centre for pediatric ophthalmology. He had also studied with Cornelius Binkhorst, the Dutch eye surgeon who pioneered lens implants in Europe. Kwitko had been on staff at the Jewish General Hospital in Montreal, but he'd quit because his chief thought his techniques were too risky and refused to permit him to perform lens implant surgery. From there, he had gone on to Bellechasse, where Duclos, an older ophthalmologist with an open mind, had found him. At St. Mary's, Duclos allowed Kwitko to perform the first intraocular lens implants in Canada. He later sent Kwitko to Moscow to learn new ways of treating myopia. When he returned, St. Mary's became the first hospital in Canada to offer the surgery.

In October, tenders were called for the addition to the hospital, even though the government had still not officially approved construction of the West Wing. In November, John Howlett stepped down after 11 years as chief of the Department of Medicine. He had been the architect of a strong department with a highly qualified staff. Upon his departure, he suggested that a subtle shift was underway at the hospital – one day soon, he said, the Catholic laity would replace nuns at St. Mary's. Guy Joron succeeded Howlett and became the first department chief with his own private office at the hospital.

On March 6, 1968, Maurice McGregor, dean of the Faculty of Medicine at McGill, recommended that St. Mary's become a teaching

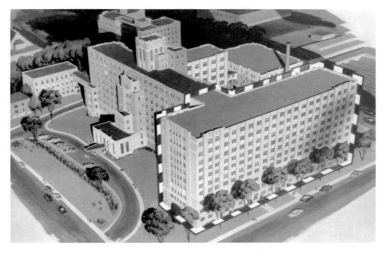

The proposed new West Wing would be built at right angles
to the old West Wing.

hospital partially affiliated with McGill for postgraduate training in anesthesia, obstetrics, gynecology, pathology, and psychiatry. Center Board president William Bennett agreed to the conditions on a two-year trial basis. It was stipulated that the chiefs of the departments involved would be jointly appointed by the university and the hospital. General surgery would be taught at the Royal Victoria, and internal medicine and orthopedics at the Montreal General. Joron then set to work to create a residency training program at St. Mary's that would be compatible with the program at the Montreal General. Because he was circumspect and always seemed to have an agenda, Joron was affectionately known around the hospital as "the Silver Fox." His smooth, efficient demeanour, however, improved hospital morale.

In spite of the hospital's precarious finances, the second phase of the St. Mary's expansion project began in April 1968 with ground-breaking for eight floors of the planned 11-storey West Wing, new underground mechanical rooms, and alterations to the powerhouse.

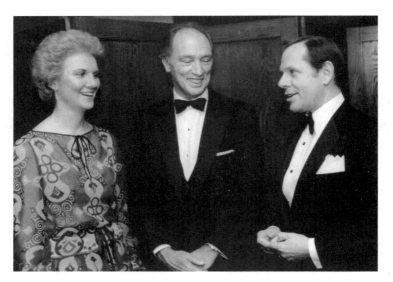

Prime Minister Pierre Elliott Trudeau was the star at the annual
St. Mary's Ball in 1968.

Again designed by Turcotte – with his firm, Agnew, Peckham and Associates – the addition had space for general laboratories, including
hematology, virology, and bacteriology, and a much larger radiology
department with 11 X-ray rooms. A second-floor surgical suite with
ten theatres was included, as well as a 12-bed intensive care unit. In addition, there was a psychiatric ward on the fourth floor, "with patient
rooms more similar to motel facilities than a standard hospital, with
a dining area, kitchenette, library, living room, television and music
rooms." Four new delivery rooms and eight labour rooms were added
to the fourth floor. The floor plans included a unique feature: "a general hallway on one side of the labour rooms, and a second hall on the
other side where mothers can exercise. Husbands will be able to join
their wives, as the corridor will connect with the father's lounge."

The caseload volume continued to soar, and the number of people
using the hospital in 1968 climbed to about 200 a day. People who
before medicare might have postponed seeing a doctor because they

couldn't afford to were now flooding the hospital. "It has become very evident that an ever-increasing number of patients who previously visited a doctor in his private office now report to a hospital emergency department," Sister Melanie noted. "Since our emergency service is not staffed by full-time medical personnel, some patients complain of having to wait long periods before being examined and treated. Measures have been taken on an experimental basis to endeavour to remedy this regrettable situation."

In the June 1968 federal election, Quebec endorsed Pierre Elliott Trudeau's promise of a just society. The Liberal Party of Canada won a majority government under its new leader, Trudeau. Six days after the election, a national, universal medicare program came into effect. Ottawa was now de facto in charge of a national scheme designed to cover all Canadians on equal terms. Benefits at last were transferable between provinces, and extra billing for services was forbidden. Trudeau's star turn at the St. Mary's Ball at the Queen Elizabeth Hotel on November 22 of that year raised $9,500 for the building fund. *Gazette* society columnist E.J. Gordon described the event as the most elegant St. Mary's Ball since the one graced by the presence of the Kennedys 14 years earlier.

But on the heels of all this gaiety came tragedy. Three weeks after the ball, the nursing school was plunged into mourning when two of its brightest students – Catherine O'Keefe, 21, and Catherine Murphy, 20 – disappeared in the woods near Ste-Adèle on December 14 while attending a religious retreat with 24 other senior nurses from the school. Their bodies were found one week later in the Doncaster River about two kilometres from the retreat house. It appeared that the two young women had gone for a walk and accidentally drowned.

CHAPTER EIGHT

A hospital should represent a mother figure. Doctors, nurses, and social workers
should never lose sight of the patient as children of infinite value…we have to
be careful to make sure a patient is never reduced to a file or a number.
~ Karl Stern

The process required to administer a health insurance plan in Quebec
was begun under duress by the Union Nationale government in
December 1969. "Either we sign and become an accomplice to an act
we find absolutely derogatory or we don't sign and deprive our citizens
of federal tax money," explained Premier Jean-Jacques Bertrand (who
had taken over from Johnson after he died suddenly of a heart attack
in 1968). But growing uncertainty over the provincial government's
intentions contributed to what St. Mary's Center Board chairman
Dennis F. Kindellan, the Quebec regional manager for Imperial Oil,
referred to as "a period of stress and uneasiness." The ongoing confusion over how and how much physicians were to be paid at St.
Mary's prompted the departure of three of the hospital's department
heads: Psychiatrist-in-Chief Noel Walsh returned to Ireland, radiologist David Shuster left for California, and chief anesthetist André Joyal
moved to Ontario.

"It is no secret, there were problems, we lost doctors, we recruited
others," Kindellan told those who attended the hospital's annual board
meeting. "Many doctors now have more patients than seems desirable,
and patients have to wait a very long time for appointments, as a result
of which they show up at the Emergency Department." Most doctors,
however, discovered that for the first time in their careers they could
count on a larger and more reliable income. Their greatest problem
was trying to accommodate the pent-up demand of thousands of people who had never before sought treatment for minor ailments.

Although the new wing was still under construction, laboratories for the Division of Clinical Immunology opened in the basement. Ihor Luhovy, a jovial if somewhat sarcastic doctor, became the department's first director. Luhovy's family had been displaced by the war, and he came to Canada from Belgium as a child. A graduate of Université de Montréal, he had specialized in immunology at the Royal Victoria before moving to St. Mary's in 1969. Under Luhovy's direction, the lab provided serological tests and conducted research into allergic and autoimmune rheumatic and collagen-vascular disease.

There had been other departmental changes that year. Jack Dinan retired as chief of surgery, and Richard Moralejo succeeded him. Jim Sullivan, a conscientious orthopedic surgeon, came on staff and introduced a new procedure for hip replacement using the McKee-Farrar prosthesis. Sullivan was joined by Carl Sutton and Len Swanson. Sutton pioneered the use of chymopapain in the treatment of sciatica, which involved injecting an enzyme from the papaya plant into spinal discs as an alternative to spinal surgery; and Swanson was an excellent, if low-key, orthopedic surgeon.

The introduction of computerized payroll accounting and a new medical records service improved efficiency. Records more than ten years old were microfilmed and the originals destroyed. In anticipation of the federal government's decision to convert to the metric system, St. Mary's became the first hospital in Canada to go metric, eight months before the legislation became law in 1970. Centigrade thermometers replaced Fahrenheit, weight scales were converted from ounces to kilograms, and a 24-hour timekeeping system was implemented. In September, the federal government contributed $3.7 million to the cost of renovating the older parts of the hospital that had been vacated when the new West Wing opened.

On December 5, 1969, St. Mary's was officially recognized by the Canadian Council on Hospital Accreditation as a teaching hospital partially affiliated with McGill University for postgraduate training in anesthesia, family medicine, general surgery, internal medicine, obstetrics and gynecology, orthopedic surgery, pathology, and psychiatry.

No formal agreement with McGill was signed, but it was generally accepted that under the arrangement, St. Mary's would remain a community-based hospital and that at least 90 percent of its primary work would be patient care. Ultra-specialized procedures such as neurosurgery, specialized pediatric surgery, cardiac surgery, and transplant surgery would be done at other McGill institutions. It took time for the magnitude of the transaction to sink in, but effectively, on the strength of a handshake, St. Mary's had taken on a dual identity as hospital and classroom. Staff doctors would be required to meet not only the requirements of St. Mary's but those of McGill as well. It also opened the hospital to a number of colourful and unorthodox McGill research specialists, such as Harry Farfan, a chain-smoker and something of a technical wizard with the human musculoskeletal structure. Like Richard Moralejo, Farfan had come from Trinidad to study at McGill, where he earned degrees in biochemistry and medicine. An enthusiastic and rambunctious surgical innovator, he introduced to orthopedic practice the Farfan facet block fusion, in which sculpted pieces were inserted into the cartilage of facet joints. Ever the iconoclast, Farfan spent 20 years researching King Kong's vertebrae as a way of discovering new ways to treat spinal disorders. "I've always had a thing about that ape," he'd chuckle. "The spine of a 40-foot ape would never have been able to support his body weight – King Kong would never have been able to get his hands off the ground, let alone climb the Empire State Building." Farfan, who died in 1994, founded the International Society for the Study of the Lumbar Spine and was active in the American College of Spine Surgeons.

Suddenly, it seemed, everyone at St. Mary's was a specialist. Finding a general practitioner to treat aches and pains was increasingly difficult. Jack Dinan was alarmed by the trend. "More and more people are making use of facilities outside the hospital as a substitute for the doctor who could and would come to their homes," he commented in his last report to the Center Board. "This makes it mandatory, I believe, to develop some kind of full-time diagnostic and emergency treatment facility manned by competent salaried medical personnel.

Remaining general practitioners would make much more efficient use of their knowledge and training. The medical life of a general practitioner would be made more attractive and we might be able to once more recruit young medical men to this presently most unattractive speciality."

By February 1970, the implications of medicare were clear. Residents and interns at 11 Montreal hospitals, including St. Mary's, who were negotiating a new contract, went on strike to back their demands for a decent salary. They had negotiated labour agreements before medicare came into effect, only to discover that their negotiated salaries exceeded the government-approved rates. Junior doctors demanded wage parity with their Ontario counterparts. Claiming that they were being exploited as cheap labour, the interns and residents walked off their jobs with the support of senior physicians and specialists, who stepped in to maintain service. Admissions were, however restricted during the three weeks it took to settle the dispute.

In May, Bill 8 changed the way physicians in Quebec were paid. Fees for services were prohibited, and doctors became, in effect, salaried government employees. That spring, a number of nursing units were transferred to the West Wing, and the wing was phased into operation over the next four months. The renal dialysis and psychiatric units opened in May, the medical units in June. After prolonged wrangling between Guy Joron, who wanted the fifth floor for chronic care patients, and Constant Nucci, who had replaced Louis James Quinn as chief of Obstetrics and Gynecology and wanted the floor for gynecology beds, it went to Nucci on the flip of a coin. He moved onto the floor in July. On July 29, Baby Lane became the first infant to be born in the new delivery rooms. The operating theatres didn't become fully operational until August. Medical residents and interns on call moved onto the fifth floor of the nurses' residence in September.

With its expanded quarters, St. Mary's became more cosmopolitan than ever. The 16 interns added to the medical staff that year represented a multitude of nationalities, including French, Egyptian, Mexican, Iranian, Irish, Chilean, Italian, and Yugoslav. But again, the hospital was aggravated by political uncertainty. A new Quebec government headed by Liberal technocrat Robert Bourassa had been elected in May on a pledge to streamline the healthcare system. Claude Castonguay ran as a Liberal candidate for a seat in the Quebec National Assembly (which he won) specifically to introduce the reforms he had recommended in a report to the previous Union Nationale government. The Department of Health and the Department of Social Welfare were rolled into one super-ministry, which took control of the Health Insurance Board, the Pension Board, and family allowances. The government also decided that the Roman Catholic Church no longer had a right to impose its institutions on the state, and, in the interim, it curtailed the plan of St. Mary's to renovate its original hospital building. The board considered the delay "a major disappointment." Then, during the first week of October, the kidnapping of the British trade commissioner, James Cross, and the abduction and murder of Quebec's labour minister, Pierre Laporte, at the hands of Front de libération du Québec terrorists, paralyzed the government's priorities, including healthcare.

The October Crisis had a detrimental effect on the St. Mary's Ball, held at the Queen Elizabeth Hotel in November. Although Governor General Roland Michener was the guest of honour at the gala celebrating the 50th anniversary of the hospital charter, tickets were a tough sell in that fraught atmosphere. Ball chairman John Pepper pleaded with the hospital's patrons (who each year accounted for 65 percent of the ball's profits) to "take a table" in order to ensure the event's success. But the ball raised only $8,000. It was one of the worst turnouts in the event's history. Crisis or no crisis, auxiliary records reflect a resolve to carry on: "Primary objective, crass motive and unpleasant to contemplate, is (1) to make money, and (2) to provide a social function so successful it will carry on in the years to come."

Due to the crisis, Quebec was the last Canadian province to join medicare, but by the second week of November, St. Mary's had processed its first claims. Enabling legislation Bill 65 established regional health councils and introduced a global system of hospital

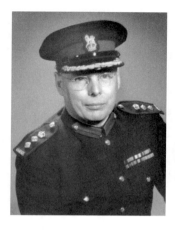

Colonel Charles Pick founded
the Oncology Unit.

budgeting. Bureaucrats now controlled hospital finances and had the
final say as to how much doctors could charge for services and how
they would be paid. The new hospital act contained more than 350
regulations largely designed to force the Church out of the hospital
business. Bill 65 surprised everyone with its scope and detail. In accord
with the new rules, the government assumed the debt St. Mary's had
incurred, it paid interns' and residents' salaries, and it standardized
nursing instruction. The contract St. Mary's had with its religious
community "was no longer relevant." Nursing education would now
be offered through the Collège d'enseignement général et profession-
nel (CEGEP) system; all applicants to the St. Mary's nursing school
would be referred to Dawson Technical College.

The implications of the legislation were staggering. For example,
hospital teaching units would be compromised if a patient insisted on
being treated by his or her own doctor and that doctor refused to par-
ticipate in the unit. "The success of the experiment will depend largely
on the cooperation of the medical staff and hospital personnel at
all levels," Sister Melanie observed. Then, on May 15, 1972, McGill's
Faculty Council renewed the trial agreement approved in 1969 to
have St. Mary's serve as a McGill University teaching hospital. The
arrangement provided new opportunities for entrepreneurial doctors;

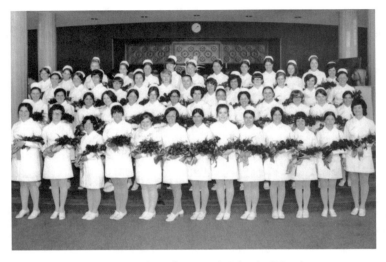

The last graduating class of St. Mary's School of Nursing, 1972.
The nurses were "a little happy, a little sad."

management had to restrain department heads engaged in empire building.

St. Mary's had to operate within a global budget. As steward of the hospital's financial well-being, the administration was hard pressed to strike a balance between what the hospital could realistically afford and enthusiasm for improved technology, increased wages, and services, which could cause operating costs to skyrocket. In spite of such obstacles, Charles Pick, who had been on staff since 1947, in partnership with a young oncologist named Peter Gruner, proposed setting up the hospital's first interdisciplinary oncology unit to coordinate the multidisciplinary care of cancer patients. Pick was a rigid, spit-and-polish army man who had served overseas with the Canadian 3rd Infantry Division during the Second World War and then became commanding officer of the 1st Canadian Medical Reserve Battalion and assistant director of medical services for the Quebec command. He enjoyed backpacking in Nepal and had little patience for the swelling administrative bureaucracy at St. Mary's.

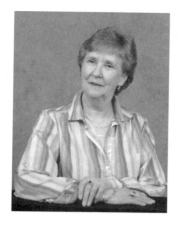

Jean Mahoney, head of the
Department of Nursing.

Gruner, Emmett Mullally's grandson, was a McGill graduate who
had come to the hospital in 1965 from Harvard University's New England Deaconess Hospital, where he had studied under James Lyman
Tullis, an internationally renowned clinical hematologist. "When I
arrived at St. Mary's, the term 'diagnostic clinic' was a euphemism
for the word 'cancer,'" Gruner recalled. "Our concern was that surgeons were doing all kinds of state-of-the-art surgery, but there was
no organized postoperative program for cancer patients." Pick and
Gruner were promoting the creation of a unit that could develop a
protocol to improve the cancer survival rate and facilitate a better
understanding of the biology of cancer, but they had to fight for it.
Developing an oncology clinic meant hiring a full-time nurse, which
Dr. Joron thought the hospital could not afford. It took a good deal of
persuasion, and there were many heated debates, but the administration relented and approved the unit. It was the first of its kind in
Montreal and the model for similar units throughout Quebec and
Canada. Hospital chaplain Jerry Sinel found a new calling and began
ministering to cancer patients in palliative care almost to the exclu-
sion of all other patients.

On Sunday, June 11, 1972, a poignant ceremony was held at École de
musique Vincent-d'Indy: 56 nurses were capped during the St. Mary's

nursing school's 43rd and final graduation exercises. They would be the last to receive their diplomas of the 1,594 nurses trained at St. Mary's since 1925. Nurses trained at the hospital had been the backbone of St. Mary's since its inception. Sister Mary Felicitas wondered aloud whether the profession could be successfully "taught at a blackboard." She couldn't help but have mixed emotions – as she told the graduates, she was "a little happy, a little relieved, a little sad." Tribute was paid to Olive Fitzgibbon, "a dedicated nurse and teacher," who, it was said, "was determined her charges would receive equal or better training than girls attending the larger hospital schools." A dispassionate account of the event is included in the records of the Sisters of Providence: "June 9-11: Final graduation ceremonies were held this weekend. With us for this occasion were Sisters Grace Maguire, Mary Felicitas, Muriel Gallagher and Sharon McCormick. The sisters attended a banquet at the Château Champlain Hotel, a tea at the nurses' residence; graduation exercises at the Vincent d'Indy School of Music, followed by a cocktail party at the Ritz-Carlton Hotel. During the festivities, a portrait of Sister M. Felicitas was unveiled."

Sister Mary Felicitas went on to St. Mary's of the Lake Hospital in Kingston, then directed the business office at St. Joseph's Auxiliary Hospital in Edmonton. She died in 2004. With the nuns gone, Marie Lund briefly took over from Sister Mary Elaine Jacobs as head of the Department of Nursing. Then Jean Mahoney, a nurse who had trained at St. Paul's Hospital in Saskatoon, Saskatchewan, and at the University of Ottawa, replaced Lund. It was Mahoney who integrated the new crop of nurses into the existing hospital culture. "It was a matter of carrying on, but it was very trial and error, especially with the first group out of the CEGEPs," she recalled. "They had the knowledge, but they didn't have the background. We had to integrate them into the hospital as practising nurses. That was a big job. But we made it work. We survived."

CHAPTER NINE

Managing a group of doctors is like herding cats. You can't herd cats.
~ Richard Moralejo

The new partnership between the Quebec government and the province's religious institutions, which had for more than a century been responsible for health and social services, brought on a maelstrom of change. Healthcare administrators, government bureaucrats, and the egos of all those who drove the system were now in play. In December 1972, the St. Mary's Hospital Foundation was established under the jurisdiction of the Minister of Financial Institutions as a separate corporate entity to raise money for the hospital and to protect its funds. Conditions regulating the investment foundation were received at the Center Board's first meeting, on February 8, 1973. Under the terms of its letters patent, the foundation was permitted "to receive gifts, grants, and contributions" to equip the hospital. Stanley Clarke, who had served so admirably as a fundraiser and as Center Board president, became the foundation's first director.

At the same time, a management troika was established to oversee the hospital. The Quebec government, in the lead position, determined the operational budget. The Center Board and the medical board, now tethered together behind the ministry with little room to manoeuvre, determined how government money would be allocated within the hospital. The changes marked a major step toward the hospital's loss of autonomy and its transformation from a Roman Catholic institution into a secular teaching institution run with much more bureaucratic zeal. Sister Melanie, turning to Richard Moralejo for help, made him the first director of Professional Services and gave

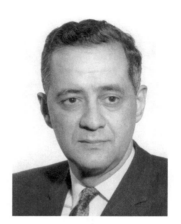

Dr. Richard Moralejo, the hospital's first
director of Professional Services.

him free reign to decide how St. Mary's would function within the
government's new regulations. Moralejo was given a mandate to "clean
up the mess." As he did not have a background in business administration, his role would be to act as a kind of master of connections, to
lubricate the bureaucratic gears and make everything mesh – the government, the medical board, the hospital administration, and the
Center Board. He likened the task of managing medical personnel to
herding cats: "You can't herd cats. They are all individuals," he said.

Moralejo approached the job of restructuring the administration
with the clear vision of the musical arranger that he was. His principal
strength was that he knew all of the players and personalities involved
and could deal with them as coequals and reconcile internal conflicts
without much fuss. Moralejo earned respect by not asking his subordinates to do anything he wouldn't do, even if it meant working the
occasional overnight emergency shift, which he did. He was the spark
plug that fired St. Mary's. By cajoling and arm-twisting, he solved
many problems and made things hum along with a minimum of
dissonance. Ben Thompson, his unflappable Jamaican friend, was
installed as surgeon-in-chief and would remain in the post for six
years. Thompson had left St. Mary's in 1955 to become an assistant resident surgeon at the Queen Mary Veterans Hospital and at the Jewish

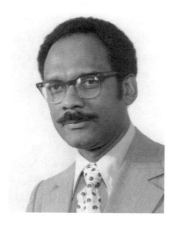

Dr. Ben Thompson, Surgeon-in-Chief.

General Hospital before moving to Northern Ontario. There he established a surgical practice in a remote community, the town of Cochrane, which had never had a surgeon before. Thompson hadn't applied for the position at St. Mary's. Moralejo, who knew him from their days together at Queen Mary Veterans, persuaded him to return to Montreal. Thompson not only got the surgeon-in-chief's job but also was awarded an assistant professorship in McGill's surgery department. The two doctors saw eye-to-eye, and Thompson often served as Moralejo's sounding board. Together they worked to make the hospital more egalitarian. Thompson encouraged the recruitment of younger surgeons, including two of his successors: John Keyserlingk and José Rodriguez.

In March 1973, in the interest of even greater efficiency, the government called upon McGill University to streamline obstetrical services in Montreal's seven English-speaking hospitals. Quebec's social affairs minister, Claude Castonguay, moved with astonishing speed to implement the university's subsequent recommendations. In May the bomb dropped: obstetrical units in three competing hospitals would be closed and consolidated at the Royal Victoria Hospital and at one other hospital, yet to be determined. The Reddy Memorial Hospital closed its unit in August, and the Catherine Booth and Queen

Elizabeth hospitals shut theirs in October. St. Mary's lost its pediatrics department, and it was widely assumed that it would also lose its obstetrics and gynecology department to the Montreal General, even though that year 1,300 babies had been delivered at St. Mary's – a 12 percent increase over the previous year. Constant Nucci, who had taken over from Louis James Quinn as head of the department in 1972, was determined to build on Quinn's legacy to make St. Mary's Montreal's major birthing centre. The objective was to have "between two and three thousand babies" delivered at the hospital each year. Nucci devoted extraordinary effort and energy to bolster the threatened department and have it do more clinical research so that it might "take advantage of the most modern and recent methods and offer obstetrical patients the best care possible." His gut instinct was that no government would take the political risk of shutting down a state-of-the-art facility that was less than three years old.

Supported by Sister Melanie, Nucci took preemptive measures to ensure that his unit stayed open. He recruited young residents, whom he "cherry-picked and screened" for their ability to fit into the hospital community. He also hired four doctors from the Reddy Memorial (including Arthur Swift, who joined Jorge Schwarz and Jack Cohen in the Division of Plastic Surgery), four from the Queen Elizabeth, and two from the Catherine Booth. New equipment, including an ultrasound machine, was acquired, and Dr. David Wisebaum, an Oxford graduate, became the hospital's first ultrasound radiologist. Stanley Skoryna began a research program on copper and zinc levels in early pregnancy, and Jozef Kaneti, a Turkish-born doctor, opened a colposcopy clinic for patients with abnormal Pap smears. Nucci also saw to it that general practitioners had privileges to deliver babies at St. Mary's and invited fathers to assist in deliveries, even those involving Caesarean sections. The hospital's infant mortality rate – 2.6 deaths for every 1,000 deliveries – was well below the provincial average of 8.3. That, especially, worked to Nucci's advantage. The government announced that the Montreal General, not St. Mary's, would lose its obstetrics and gynecology department.

If St. Mary's was to remain indispensable as a community hospital, it also had to enhance its commitment to family medicine and provide general ambulatory care. Constance Lapointe, an endocrinologist, was invited to establish a family medicine department. Originally from Ohio, Lapointe had obtained her medical degree from the Women's Medical College of Pennsylvania in Philadelphia and had worked in Washington, D.C., before moving to Canada in 1962.

"What struck me at the time was that everyone on staff was becoming overtrained, in a way," Lapointe recalled. "From a medical standpoint, it was wonderful to have all this training, but no one wanted to do family medicine anymore." Peter O'Shaunessey, then in his seventies, certainly did. O'Shaunessey had no intention of retiring, and he worked in the new department as an extremely valuable preoperative physician. Although Lapointe encountered some resistance, the Department of Family Medicine opened on the second floor of the former nurses' residence in 1974. Family doctors Linda Riven, Harvey Halperin, and Charles Pierce were added as full-time teachers and clinicians.

In 1924, when the hospital was founded, doctors didn't need much education in order to practise. By the 1950s, they not only required a university degree but also an additional three to seven years of residency training in a specialized field of practice, such as pediatrics, surgery, or neurology. But by the mid-1970s, even this level of preparation was inadequate to meet the complex demands encountered in new areas, such as laparoscopic surgery, pediatric metabolic disorders, or critical care. To accommodate the growing demand for super-specialists who had practised in one narrow field until they were better at it than anyone else, the Collège des médecins du Québec and the Royal College of Physicians and Surgeons of Canada decreed that all postgraduate training had to be offered under the aegis of a university. Any remaining objections to an affiliation with McGill were now academic. Lingering reservations on both sides were resolved, and the university was authorized to name a representative of its own to the hospital board. McGill picked John Howlett, who was on staff at both

St. Mary's and McGill. His appointment did not result in any appreciable changes to existing hospital privileges or procedures.

With the completion of the West Wing in 1975, the hospital now boasted the most modern facilities of their type in Montreal. But the expansion brought on a major parking headache. There was talk of building a two-level underground parking garage between the old nursing school and the playground, which would ease the parking problem and bring in additional revenue. But the Center Board did not warm to the idea. Instead, the hospital's front lawn was paved over and turned into a parking lot.

A new, expanded library with books from the collections of Hingston and H.R. Gray was opened on the library's 25th anniversary. Lucile Lavigueur's efforts to improve the quality of the library's services was recognized by the Canadian Council on Hospital Accreditation, which commended Lavigueur for the library's "well-planned facilities, good organization, well-balanced collection, and wide scope of material." The library continued to expand, and so did its staff. Marjolaine Martel, who is still at St. Mary's, was hired as a library technician in 1983 and worked for nine years with another technician, Guylaine Choquette-Paulin. When Lavigueur retired, in 1988, she was replaced by Jeannine Lawlor, who ran the library until Gilles Teasdale took over from her in 2003.

Dr. Gaston Duclos, who had built ophthalmology into a full department in 1971, died in an automobile accident in 1976. His assistant, Dr. Kurt Schirmer, a native of Baden bei Wien, Austria, succeeded him. Schirmer had studied at the University of Vienna, and, after coming to Canada in 1953, he had interned at the Jeffery Hale Hospital in Quebec City. He went on to study ophthalmology at the University of Toronto and was an eye surgeon at St. Joseph's Hospital in Sudbury, Ontario, where he successfully implanted an anterior chamber lens, before coming to St. Mary's to work with Duclos. As department head, Schirmer went out on a limb by sending Marvin Kwitko to New York to train with Charles Kelman, the developer of phacoemulsification, a technique that used ultrasonic waves to emulsify the nucleus of the

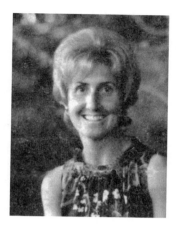

Dr. Constance Lapointe, first Chief,
Department of Family Medicine.

lens of the eye, making it possible to remove cataracts without removing the lens, which until then had been standard practice. Kwitko
brought the technique to St. Mary's, and patients thus treated could
go home the day after surgery instead of spending ten days in hospital. To support the volume of such eye operations, it became necessary
to introduce day surgery, then a controversial idea; the practice was
eventually accepted, to the benefit of all hospital departments. Kwitko
became head of the Department of Ophthalmology in 1994, and he
remained a high-profile doctor until he died, in 2002. He was succeeded by W.E.S. Connolly and Conrad Kavalec, who is now in charge.

In 1978, St. Mary's was asked to conform to the Charter of the French
Language (Bill 101) by adding a French version to its name, which was
then St. Mary's Hospital. At the Center Board meeting of April 26,
1978, the board adopted a special bylaw to add the name Centre hospitalier de St-Mary and to change the English version to St. Mary's
Hospital Center. This special bylaw was also ratified by the Board of
Governors.

Costs associated with universal healthcare continued to escalate.
The government ignored inflation and bargained wages, yet it also
began insisting that the hospital implement cost-cutting measures.

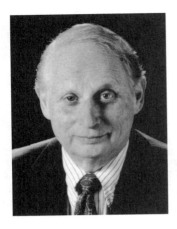

Dr. Marvin Kwitko pioneered
lens implant surgery.

St. Mary's was forced to cope with unrealistic financial constraints. Robert Grassby, who had a strong sense of business acumen, was brought in to chair the Center Board. As president of Montreal Loco-motive Works, Grassby had once successfully defied a United States government ban and sold locomotives to Cuba. Grassby's biggest headache was triggered by the 1976 election of René Lévesque and his separatist Parti Québécois (PQ). "Castro I could deal with – I knew what to expect," he said. "Lévesque proved to be more of a challenge. With the election of the PQ, St. Mary's no longer had anyone we knew in government. There was no one we could pick up the phone and call in Quebec City. It was a whole new ball game."

With the establishment of its interdisciplinary research unit, St. Mary's had begun receiving grants from pharmaceutical companies and the Department of Health and Welfare. Then, in 1977, the Parti Québécois introduced its Régie régionale de la santé, a province-wide network of 16 administrative health regions. In theory, the idea was to decentralize administration; in practice, it entrenched a new level of bureaucrats and bean counters who were far removed from the prac-tical aspects of running a hospital. The introduction of Bill 101 officially put an end to bilingualism in Quebec and put a French face on all Quebec government institutions, including hospitals. The bill's

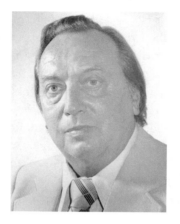

Bill Busat succeeded Sister Melanie as chief administrator.

Section 28 stipulated that St. Mary's would have five years to provide service in French to all patients. Just how the law was to be applied was open to interpretation. In a parallel move, the government set up the Commission de surveillance de la langue française, whose job it was to monitor violations of the language law. Sister Melanie, nearing retirement, had never been fluently bilingual, and, at 64, she was not about to become so. Seeing the writing on the wall, she quit as the hospital's chief executive officer. "Government control of hospitals has gone far enough," she told the *Montreal Star*, "but it is natural for the control to lie where the money comes from. The problem is, I resent it when the government tells us what has to be done then doesn't supply the money to allow us to do it. There is less satisfaction, less creativity and less chance to solve problems on one's own."

Bill Busat, who had been Sister Melanie's assistant for 20 years, replaced her. Busat was a coal-miner's son from Gelsenkirchen, Germany. He had studied business at the University of Munich, but when Hitler threatened to redraw the map of Europe, he had gone to work for the Office of Strategic Services, a US intelligence agency. During the Second World War, he had been a spy for the American Army, and he'd worked in intelligence in the postwar reconstruction period. When the war ended, Busat moved to New York and took a post as assistant comptroller for the North Central Bronx Hospital before joining St. Mary's in 1957 as director of finance. In the early 1960s, Sister Melanie sent him to Winnipeg to study hospital management at the University of Manitoba. Busat was also cofounder and vice president of the Institut des contrôleurs et des comptables d'hôpitaux de la province de Québec. He didn't adapt easily to the promotion. Busat could be a rather pompous man; he was often condescending and sometimes made his subordinates' lives difficult, but he was undeniably good at what he did. The character of Everett Kingsley, administrator of the fictional St. Paul's Hospital in Peter Clement's roman à clef *Lethal Practice*, is a thinly disguised depiction of Busat. Clement refers to "a vigorous administrator who had become increasingly devoted to the three martini lunch long after the rest of the world had given it up." Although Busat ran the hospital for the next six years, he depended heavily on his director of Financial Services, Oswald Schmidt, and on his director of Professional Services, Richard Moralejo. "Busat was one hell of a sharp cookie," said one staff member. "He was influential, and I think part of the secret of his success was that he completely bamboozled his board of directors. He didn't always tell the Center Board what it needed to know."

The hospital began replacing its unilingual staff, and by 1978, Busat was satisfied that St. Mary's was sufficiently bilingual to treat French-speaking patients in their own language. Most healthcare professionals on staff had a working knowledge of French, but few knew it well enough to pass the government's exacting oral and written language proficiency tests. The hospital's surgeon-in-chief, Ben Thompson, for example, had been taking French classes twice a week. Though he could communicate "reasonably well" with his French-speaking patients, he found himself intimidated by the Quebec government inspectors who began showing up at the hospital. Reluctantly, Thompson gave up his position and moved to Kincardine, Ontario. José Rodriguez, an amiable Spaniard who had come to St. Mary's as an intern in 1965, stepped into his shoes. Born in Valencia during the Spanish Revolution, Rodriguez, son of a private detective in the

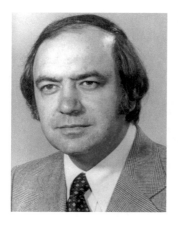

Dr. José Rodriguez performed the first
liver resection at St. Mary's.

Republican government, had known from the age of 13 that he wanted
to be a doctor. "My father had a friend who was a surgeon who was
my idol," he recalled. "But later, as a medical student at the University
of Madrid, I realized he was not such a hot surgeon after all." Before
Thompson resigned, Rodriguez had considered leaving Quebec because of the language climate, but in the end he chose to stay on.

Rodriguez trained with Jack Dinan. The turning point in his career
came when Dinan's son needed surgery and Rodriguez was the only
one Dinan trusted to perform the operation. A confident, highly
efficient surgeon, Rodriguez performed the first liver resection at
St. Mary's in 1976, and he was flattered to be invited to become the
hospital's surgeon-in-chief. The appointment also entailed his being
made associate professor of surgery at McGill University. By then,
Guy Joron had been named the university's director of continuing
medical education, and, with Constant Nucci's appointment as McGill's
associate dean of postgraduate education and associate professor of
obstetrics and gynecology, it was apparent that doctors from St. Mary's
were becoming entrenched at the university. In 1979, McGill brought
in Mark Yaffe, an engaging young doctor with a master's degree in
clinical science in family medicine, to enhance the department at

St. Mary's. Yaffe was born in Deep River, Ontario. His father was a nuclear radiation chemist who led the Canadian delegation to the first Atoms for Peace conference in Geneva in the mid-1950s and later served as chairman of the Department of Chemistry at McGill. Yaffe grew up in Montreal. After being schooled briefly in Vienna, he received his medical degree from McGill in 1976. A W.K. Kellogg fellowship holder, Yaffe was the only trainee to design his own study program at the two Canadian universities that offered Kellogg programs: McGill and the University of Western Ontario. His master's thesis concentrated on the 11 developmental tasks associated with the so-called midlife crisis and explored how family doctors might best deal not only with such issues as physiological changes but also with retirement, financial planning, and overall quality of life for the elderly.

In February 1980, James "Big Jim" Sullivan, director of the hospital's orthopedic division, went off to serve as chief medical officer at the Lake Placid Winter Olympics in New York State. When the games were over, he opened a sports medicine clinic at St. Mary's to evaluate and treat injured athletes, but it was soon curtailed due to budget constraints. The hospital's renovated Emergency Department opened in October 1980, a surgical day centre was established, and it seemed the administration had at last adjusted to the rhythms of the new management regime. Brian O'Neill, the executive vice president of the National Hockey League, had replaced Grassby as chairman of the Center Board in 1976. He didn't anticipate any further problems in dealing with the government. "Finances were always a major problem," O'Neill remembers, "but we negotiated with the banks to pay off our overhead, and we kept close to our budgets. Bill Busat had established a good rapport with Quebec City; Oswald Schmidt understood the new system of Régies régionales and was very accurate about our obligations to the government. Our staff was in good shape, we had good chiefs, and Richard Moralejo was a consummate diplomat. The foundation was starting to raise funds for the hospital. More and more, a lot of French was spoken around the building. We had a lot of French-speaking patients, and we treated patients in French. But we still thought of ourselves as an English-speaking Irish Catholic institution. We had no idea what we were in for."

On March 19, 1981, Marie-Marthe Larose, a 67-year-old housewife, was admitted to St. Mary's for an emergency throat cancer operation. While Larose was in intensive care, her family had nothing but effusive praise for her irrepressible surgeon, John Keyserlingk, and for the quality of medical care she received. Keyserlingk was the youngest of five children of a Prussian count, who had come to Montreal just before the Second World War. His father had worked as a journalist with British United Press in Europe, converted to Catholicism, and then moved to Montreal, where he edited the *Ensign*, a short-lived national Catholic newspaper that was based in the city. His son John was born at St. Mary's in 1947 and was schooled in French at Collège Brébeuf; he received his medical degree from Université de Montréal in 1972. Larose, who had been in a coma for much of her time in the hospital, died on May 8, and her daughter, Huguette, decided to file a complaint against Keyserlingk with Quebec's French-language watchdog, the Commission de surveillance de la langue française. In it she claimed that the hospital had violated Bill 101, because the doctor and three nurses had spoken English to each other while treating her mother; for this reason, Marie-Marthe Larose had not been able to die peacefully in French. While it is impossible to attribute motives – which could have been prompted by genuine grief or by a mischievous political agenda – it is true that six months earlier, the Quebec government had lost its first independence referendum, and Huguette was married to a high-profile Quebec separatist, Paul Guy, chairman of Quebec's securities commission – Autorité des marchés financiers – and a former president of the PQ's Notre-Dame-de-Grace riding association. The subsequent government investigation into the highly publicized complaint contributed to a chapter in the hospital's history that was blackly comic, infuriating, and at times downright silly. The central issue was this: Did nurses speaking English to each other disquiet an unconscious patient who might still have heard them and not understood what they were saying? Jack Dinan remarked, "Any

Catholic I ever saw dying doesn't care whether they hear either English or French. All they want to hear is Latin" (the language once used to administer sacraments to the dying). The case dragged on for the better part of two years, and it poisoned the civil atmosphere in Quebec. "It was an unfortunate situation with unfortunate consequences," says Keyserlingk. "I had been schooled thoroughly in French, went through medical school in French, and it was obvious that when I testified in French before the commission that Huguette Larose had not done her homework. I was married to a francophone and my children didn't speak one word of English until I went to study at the Royal Marsden Hospital in London. I thought that was amusing."

A government investigator with neither medical nor legal expertise examined the shift schedules and arrived at a bureaucratic conclusion, as only bureaucrats can: While Larose was at St. Mary's, she was subjected to English 34 percent of the time. He would later concede, however, that the staff in the intensive care unit spent most of their time in silence; they were occupied with monitoring life-support systems. While all of this was going on, the administration continued to make internal appointments on the basis of medical competence, not linguistic ability. Ironically, in October 1982, when the fluently bilingual Guy Joron retired as chief of the Department of Medicine, his protégé, Peter McCracken, who spoke what he calls "hospital French," replaced him. McCracken was only 35, but he was already recognized as a specialist in geriatric care and had been named coordinator of geriatric medicine at McGill University. McCracken had been schooled at Loyola College and had obtained his medical degree from McGill in 1970. He did his resident training in internal medicine at the University of Alberta before coming to St. Mary's in 1976. Joron steered McCracken into working with aging patients, then sent him to England for formal training in geriatric care. As chief of the Department of Medicine, McCracken was preoccupied with building McGill University's Division of Geriatric Medicine. The introduction of geriatric care at St. Mary's meant a reduction in the number of acute care beds;

and, because geriatric care took beds away from the surgery department, the hospital now needed fewer surgical residents. To lessen the impact, chief surgeon Ben Thompson encouraged the early discharge of patients who had undergone major surgery.

The language issue continued to take its toll on hospital morale. The chief of Anesthesia, himself a francophone, left St. Mary's in disgust. "It was an unhappy time for some individuals at the hospital," acknowledged McCracken. "But, frankly, the language controversy really had little impact on the day-to-day operations of my department. The issue received media attention, but within the hospital, as far as patients were concerned, everything went along blissfully as it always did. We didn't go out of our way to antagonize the government, and we tried to pacify the bureaucrats as much as that was possible at the time."

Jean Mahoney stepped down as director of Nursing Services and moved to Ontario. Her assistant, Helene McCormack, took over the department. McCormack, raised in Drummondville, had a French-Canadian mother and an English father. A product of the St. Mary's School of Nursing, she had studied at the University of Ottawa and had been Mahoney's assistant director of nursing since 1973.

For at least three years, Constant Nucci, too, had been increasingly uncomfortable with the Quebec political situation and the government's ongoing refusal to buy new equipment for his department. Even though he was by now also associate dean of postgraduate medical education at McGill, he resigned as head of Obstetrics and Gynecology and moved to Toronto to take up the same post at St. Michael's Hospital. "I was bored with teaching, and I was happy with what I had achieved at St. Mary's, and I thought it was time to bring in new blood," he explained. Nucci was replaced by David Schaffelburg, a Nova Scotia-born doctor who had grown up in Montreal and who had been a resident at St. Mary's in the 1970s while he was studying medicine at McGill. Shaffelburg quickly became frustrated with the government's indifference to the hospital's requirements. "The biggest problem we had was that there was never enough money to buy the essential equipment we needed," he said. "We had a report saying all our fetal monitors were obsolete and should be scrapped, and we had to keep working with the old monitors because there was never any money to replace them."

Ironically, as the language controversy raged, Quebec's healthcare and social services ministry awarded St. Mary's its Prix Persillier-Lachapelle. The award recognized the hospital's achievement in developing its family medicine department and in providing new alternatives to hospitalization while at the same time maintaining high standards of patient care.

The 90-page report issued by the language commission on March 8, 1983 ruled, predictably, that Madame Larose had not been treated in French to the government's satisfaction, and the commission threatened to slap the hospital with a $1,000 fine. St. Mary's was given four months to ensure that French-language services were available "all the time and to everyone who has a right to it."

Center Board president John Pepper tersely replied that St. Mary's would not conform to the directive. Pepper, a scrappy lawyer and son-in-law of the architect who designed St. Mary's, filed an appeal. He found support for his intransigence in the editorial pages of French and English newspapers. *Le Soleil* leapt to the defense of St. Mary's: "Young people have excellent reasons for wanting to leave Quebec... with such an obvious attack on a hospital, Quebec nationalism shows a baneful stubbornness under the circumstances." *Le Devoir* noted that while "the character of English language institutions is certainly changed by the government's language policy, it would be an exaggeration to claim that the policy requires everyone who works in a hospital to have a knowledge of French." The *Gazette* was much more blunt: "The renewed attack on St. Mary's falls like a boor's obscenity into the civilized dialogue lately developing on language relations in Quebec. As long as French services are generally available in an English institution, there is no requirement for every single employee to have any more knowledge of French than is necessary for his or her particular task."

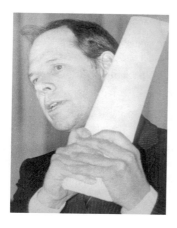

John Pepper, president of the Board of Directors, fought the Quebec government over its language policy.

Everyone rallied around St. Mary's. The staff endorsed the hospital, removing their name tags so that no one could identify their ethnic backgrounds. Richard French, Westmount's member of the provincial National Assembly, donated his MNA salary increase to help finance the hospital's court battle. In the legislature, the Liberal opposition introduced a motion of nonconfidence in the Parti Québécois government, blaming Premier René Lévesque for reneging on his promise to protect the right of English-speaking Quebecers to their own institutions.

In the midst of the uproar, St. Mary's embarked on a five-year, $10 million capital campaign to complete two floors of the West Wing, rebuild the front entrance, and expand the radiology department. Sean Harty, an eloquent, cerebral high school teacher with a degree in counselling psychology from the State University of New York, was hired to direct the campaign. The son of Irish immigrants, Harty had grown up in St-Henri. He had initially taken the job on a contract basis out of a sense of social responsibility. "What attracted me was that it was a fundraiser for our community's hospital and for our family's hospital," he said. "I was an idealist, interested in organizational behaviour in management, and I wanted to contribute something to the community." Harty had no experience in raising money. "The board really stepped on the sea on that one," he conceded. He was to find, however, that the publicity arising from the language brouhaha would attract substantial donations from both French and English corporate sponsors. The fundraising drive was fuelled by public testimonials, including one from a 76-year-old British visitor, with the rather suspect name of John Henry, who was quoted as saying that never in his life had he "witnessed such efficiency, thoroughness, and compassion in a medical staff" as he had at St. Mary's. And Harty discovered that he enjoyed working at the hospital more than he did teaching. In his own words, he "became addicted to St. Mary's."

The hospital also brought in a public relations director, Barbara Brown Bourke, to deal with the media and to launch a bilingual hospital newsletter – *It's Happening at St. Mary's*. Brown was charged with helping to wean the hospital away from its image as a Roman Catholic institution, and, as a result, she had to withstand more than a decade of criticism.

By late 1983, the coercive aspects of Bill 101 had become so unpopular that the bill's author, Camille Laurin, was replaced in Lévesque's Cabinet by Gérald Godin, a poet and a democrat who stood head and shoulders above nationalist partisan politics. As the government's new minister responsible for the application of Quebec's language laws, Godin urged hard-line language commissioners to either be more open to the sensitivities of English-speaking Quebecers or quit. "There may be hawks at the commission, but they have to realize a dove is in charge now," he said. "They will have to act like doves too, or get out."

There were changes at the Center Board level as well. The fiery John Pepper was succeeded as board president by the far less confrontational Patrick Rourke. Robert Grassby, who had been president of the Center Board in the mid-1970s, took over from Stanley Clarke as president of the St. Mary's Hospital Foundation. In the end, cooler heads prevailed. Godin sensibly intervened. On December 21, 1983, Quebec's Justice Department advised the language commission that it had no grounds to take St. Mary's to court because it would be impossible to prove that the hospital had not taken "fair and reasonable measures" to ensure that the patient had been served in French. The same day, section 25 of Bill 101, which required that services in French be fully available as of January 1, 1984, was abolished; as long as French-language services were generally available in an English-speaking institution, the government would not require everyone on staff to speak French. With that, the wave of outrage that had been building subsided.

Some, in fact, have suggested that these events actually kept the government from closing St. Mary's 10 years later. "As a result of the language issue, we got to know people in government we wouldn't have otherwise known, and they got to know us," said Patrick Wickham, who was secretary of the Center Board at the time. "It worked to our advantage. When the PQ began closing hospitals in 1993, they didn't dare touch us. By then they knew who we were. The government didn't want to go through the same political headache all over again."

CHAPTER TEN

A hospital can't be a little bit of everything, doing everything for everyone all the time. Doctors have to realize that not all departmental chiefs are equal.
~ Constant Nucci

In 1984, St. Mary's marked its 60th anniversary with what that year's annual report described as "steady progress and rising confidence." On the surface, there appeared to be every reason for self-congratulation. St. Mary's was well on its way to achieving its $10 million fundraising objective, and the new obstetrics and gynecology clinic had opened in the hospital annex. The practice of having the same nurse take care of both mother and newborn was introduced, enhancing continuity of care and security for mother and child. The new peripheral vascular diagnostic laboratory under the direction of Carl Émond opened, and efforts were underway to reorganize the second floor to house more intermediate care patients. Volunteer Lil Parsons set up a card table and began selling second-hand books, an enterprise that would eventually expand into a lobby boutique and bring substantial revenues to the hospital auxiliary.

St. Mary's was busier than ever. It was operating at full occupancy, and outpatient visits continued to increase. But there were disturbing undercurrents. Even though the Ministry of Health and Social Services kept approving expanded services and specialized medical equipment, it stubbornly refused to cover the higher operating costs they entailed. As a result of chronic government underfunding, the hospital was $2.3 million over budget. Government-funded medicare continued to afford excellent care for most patients, but, 15 years into the program, there was an uncomfortable cash squeeze as the demand

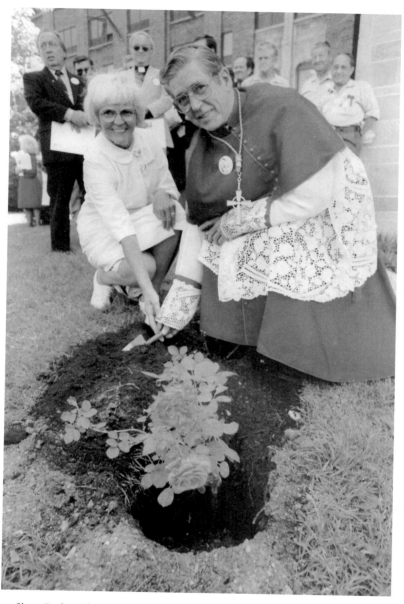

Sister Evelyn O'Grady and Bishop Leonard Crowley plant the "Pope's roses" to mark the hospital's 60th anniversary.

for healthcare services, combined with expensive advances in medical technology, outstripped the government's willingness to pay.

Of course, St. Mary's was not the only hospital in financial straits. Faced with a healthcare funding crisis, the government did what governments always do in such circumstances: it appointed a committee to undertake a detailed survey of the strengths and weaknesses of Quebec's 60 biggest health centres. Overcrowding was becoming an even greater problem, but St. Mary's seemed to be one of the few hospitals in the city that was managing to juggle the admitting, processing, and discharging of patients. "I operated on the principle that no bed in the hospital was sacred, and emergency cases came first," said Richard Moralejo, director of Professional Services. "My philosophy was that every department had to share a bit of the suffering, and if you pulled one log out of the jam, things would start to move. If I had to, I'd cancel a surgery and admit an emergency case instead."

The hospital's diamond jubilee coincided with another significant event: Pope John Paul II's three-day visit to Montreal on his first tour of Canada. To honour the Pope, a new rose hybrid was developed, and 60 of "the Pope's bushes" – one for each year of the hospital's existence – were planted that spring in front of the building.

Physicians are a well-connected fraternity, but perhaps no doctor at St. Mary's was as well connected as immunologist Andy Gutkowski. He came to work with Ihor Luhovy, who had established the Division of Clinical Immunology and Rheumatology at St. Mary's in 1969. The division offered serological tests, then a relatively new medical specialty. In addition to providing services for the hospital, the two doctors were involved in drug trials. Gutkowski, like the Pope, was of Polish heritage. Born in Vilnius, Lithuania, he had studied medicine at Trinity College, Dublin. He moved to Canada in 1960, settling first in Winnipeg, where he joined a general practice group. Eventually, he decided to pursue a career in internal medicine, starting the program at St. Boniface Hospital and completing it at the Montreal General in 1971. Among Gutkowski's acquaintances was a doctor who had treated the Pope following the assassination attempt that occurred in St.

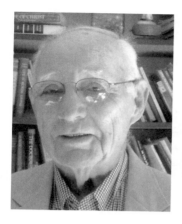

Dr. Gerald Berry fought for
a new autopsy suite.

Peter's Square in 1981. Gutkowski had met the pontiff in Rome. When
the Pope arrived in Montreal in September, he dispatched his private
secretary, Stanislaw Dziwisz, to call on Gutkowski and to visit one of
Gutkowski's patients at the hospital. Dziwisz went on to become
Archbishop of Krakow, and, in 2006, he was made a cardinal by Bene-
dict XVI.

David Kahn stepped down as chief pathologist in 1984, and Gerald
Berry succeeded him. A strapping, avuncular doctor affectionately
known as "The Bear," Berry was a civil servant's son who had grown
up in Westmount. Inspired by Richard Llewellyn's tales of hardship in
Wales, he decided to go into medicine. Berry first came to St. Mary's as
a resident in 1963, four years after obtaining his medical degree from
St. Francis Xavier University, where Norman McLetchie had been one
of his professors. Berry went into private practice in Rosemère, but,
with a family of five to support, he quickly arrived at the conclusion
that he was "heading nowhere as a GP." Encouraged and influenced by
Kahn, whom he considered his intellectual mentor, Berry studied at
McGill to be a pathologist. He then became director of laboratories at
the Lakeshore General Hospital before taking over the pathology
department at St. Mary's in 1982. Berry took up his duties just as the
hospital had begun to notice a resurgence of tuberculosis, which had

been transmitted by immigrants arriving from Vietnam. At the same time, a mysterious respiratory infection was afflicting several male patients. Doctors like Joe Dylewski, a microbiologist who had just returned from studying in Africa and California, were intrigued by the new illness, which seemed to be targeting homosexuals. "Something was happening. We recognized it as a sort of strain of HTLV – human T-cell lymphotropic virus – but the viral nature of acquired immune deficiency, or AIDS, had not yet been determined," Dylewski recalled. "We weren't being inundated with cases, but we saw some of it then."

In order to diagnose tuberculosis and deal more efficiently with other respiratory diseases, Berry wanted to buy a Bach-Tech machine, which could process cases in six hours instead of two or three weeks. But each time he submitted an application for the instrument, it was rejected. "It was really bloody awful," Berry recalled. "The hospital was subject to tremendous bureaucratic incompetence. The government's refusal to approve the machine was unacceptable, knowing it was available. We applied for it. Refused. We applied again. Refused. Third time. Refused. But this time the head of the government committee that OK'd medical equipment came to the hospital. The stuffed shirt sat down with us and said, 'Don't you people know that when we apply for equipment, the government requires you to supply us with a list of tenders with two or three quotes from competitors?' We looked at him and said, 'As someone who is supposed to know what you're doing, don't you know there is only one manufacturer of this machine? One price? Bach-Tech has no competitors.'"

At the same time, Peter Duffy took over as chief of the Emergency Department and tried to provide good care under trying circumstances. Duffy was born in Perth, Ontario, and raised in Winnipeg. He studied medicine at Queen's University and also completed a degree in literature and philosophy. From there he went to work at the addiction research facility at the Kingston Psychiatric Hospital, then did a two-year stint with the National Film Board of Canada, where he supervised a project at Collins Bay Penitentiary using video cameras to promote prison reform. At St. Mary's, Duffy trained as an intern, working in the outpatient department. "Emergency is the gatekeeper of the hospital, and it was clear by then that there was no room within the hospital beyond the gates," Duffy said. "The actual impact of closing one or two beds on every floor was not all that great, but the accumulated impact on emergency was overwhelming." There was no quick fix to any of the mounting problems. In September, a Progressive Conservative government was elected in Ottawa on a program of deficit reduction. The new prime minister, Brian Mulroney, vowed to "adjust Canadian expectations to government largesse," including healthcare.

Mulroney was invited to be guest of honour at the St. Mary's 60th Anniversary Ball. He sent his new minister of justice, John Crosbie, in his place. In its first budget, Mulroney's government implemented some of the harshest cost-cutting measures the provinces and municipalities had ever had to bear. That meant even less money for healthcare, and spending restraint at all levels of government became the order of the day. The residency program atrophied – it went from having a full-time staff of four at various stages of training to nil – but the workload continued to intensify. As a result, the harmonious atmosphere in the laboratories was eroded. Residents who had been without a contract for three years started working to rule, then they staged a one-day strike to demand wage parity with their counterparts in Ontario. Doctors performing autopsies found themselves working in primitive conditions – Gerald Berry described "a cold, windowless space of bare concrete and stainless steel made colder by a network of exposed steam and water pipes snaking in and out of the walls, which themselves were dull with old, chipped paint." The room wasn't ventilated, and in the summer, pathologists had to work in temperatures of about 38 degrees Celsius with the doors to the refrigeration room left open and electric fans running. For the next 10 years, Berry lobbied to get a new suite built on the second floor of the powerhouse facing St. Joseph's Oratory. "Those years were really bloody awful," he says.

"When the government cut the budget, you translated the cuts and cut people and services accordingly. As soon as you cut the people, the government came in and complained about it."

In March 1985, the hospital's Council of Physicians and Dentists recommended that St. Mary's ban smoking on the premises; St. Mary's followed the lead of several other Montreal hospitals, putting the ban into effect in September. While St. Mary's was expected to keep abreast of the latest medical advances and acquire expensive state-of-the-art equipment, the government eliminated medical training programs to cut costs. Still, hospitals were expected to operate on less money. McGill University, caught in the cash crunch, reduced its teaching programs for specialty residents at the senior level. That caused concern at the hospital. "We felt it was important to have a proper balance between the top and the bottom of the hierarchy of our clinical teaching units," said Richard Moralejo. Acute nursing shortages complicated matters. In 1985, the hospital admitted 16,000 patients – a 3 percent increase over the previous year – but because of chronic staff shortages, in the winter of 1985, it was forced to close one of its nursing units for a month.

Bill Busat retired in 1986 after nine years as director general. Constant Nucci came back from Toronto in June to replace him. Nucci was the first doctor in the hospital's history to fill the position, and he returned to St. Mary's with good will in reserve. His stewardship as chief of Obstetrics and Gynecology had been inspirational, and he was also remembered fondly for serving as chairman of the St. Mary's education committee and its Council of Physicians and Dentists.

Doctors on staff generally welcomed his return, believing that as a fellow physician, Nucci would empathize with them, understand their grievances, and champion their causes. One of Nucci's first official duties as head of the hospital was to attend the auxiliary's gala evening at the Montreal Museum of Fine Arts, in January 1987, which had been organized to inaugurate the exhibition *Vatican Splendour: Masterpieces of Baroque Art*. The papal nuncio to Canada, Angelo Palmas, and Montreal's auxiliary bishop, Leonard Crowley, opened the exhibition.

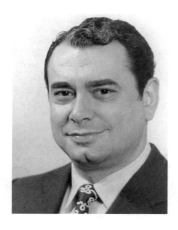

Dr. Constant Nucci, the first doctor
to be named CEO of St. Mary's.

The St. Mary's Auxiliary, under the direction of Dr. Hingston's grand-
daughter, Janet Macklem, sponsored the show. The funds raised
enabled the auxiliary to make a record-breaking annual donation to
the hospital foundation of $250,000. It would be the first and last time
Nucci would be able to relax on the job.

Nucci had been gone for three years, but he knew what he was coming back to, and he was apprehensive. He ran into difficulties almost
from the start. Managing an entire hospital would present a far greater
challenge than running a single department within it. The government
directives St. Mary's received were contradictory, and Nucci found
himself trying to satisfy the requirements of a government-managed
healthcare system while juggling the conflicting demands of his fellow doctors and department heads. He introduced what he thought
would be a more proactive approach to administration, and in this he
would depend heavily on his director of Professional Services, Richard
Moralejo, for support. Moralejo had once been Nucci's superior, and
he probably knew more about St. Mary's than anyone. Now the roles
were reversed, and as Nucci worked to bring about change, it soon
became apparent that he and Moralejo had competing philosophies
and different management styles. Corporate success stories often feature dominant personalities, and Nucci, not shy about leading with his

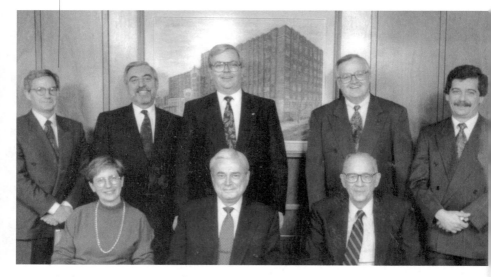

Senior Management, 1986. [Front row, left to right] Helene McCormack, Director of Nursing, Dr. Constant Nucci, Chief Executive Officer, Dr. Richard Moralejo, Director of Professional Services. [Back row, left to right] Ron Newham, Director of Human Resources, Harold Thuringer, Director of St. Mary's Hospital Foundation, Terrence Meehan, Director of Technical Services, Sean Harty, Assistant Executive Director, Larry English, Director of Finance.

chin, soon found himself embroiled in conflicts with a number of department heads, including Moralejo, over the hospital's future.

One of Nucci's first challenges was to come up with a strategic "plan d'équilibre budgétaire" to cope with the government's assigned budget. "I was fully conscious of my proper background and my competence to handle the medical and linguistic aspects of the job, but my big anxiety was that I can barely make change for a dollar," he admitted. "My knowledge of hospital finances was limited, and I made no bones about it. But suddenly I had to see the entire operation from an administrative point of view, not just from the medical side of things. It was fascinating to see the operation from a non-doctor point of view." One of his first tasks was to sort out some erroneous billing in the psychiatry department. Medicare had been substantially over-billed for work by professionals who didn't qualify. As it turned out, the rules governing billing were ambiguous, and the matter was resolved when the government agreed to split the difference with the hospital.

After years of negotiation with the authorities, St. Mary's acquired its first computed axial tomography (CT scan) machine. It went into operation in July 1987. The medical imaging device could capture a series of three-dimensional images of the body very quickly. St. Mary's forged an agreement with the Queen Elizabeth Hospital permitting that hospital to refer four or five patients a week to St. Mary's for CT scans, which brought St. Mary's an additional $90,000 a year. Other sophisticated state-of-the-art equipment was installed, including a new defibrillator for intensive care, four pulse oximeters, a 16-channel electroencephalograph, and a new infant care system. Ralph Dadoun, a research assistant at the Montreal Neurological Institute, was brought in to reorganize the laboratories and make them more cost-effective. The government had not increased the hospital's budget base since 1972. Due to chronic underfunding, Nucci and the Center Board found themselves confronting a $1.9 million deficit. Nucci was forced to close 30 beds, which increased waiting times for elective surgery, placed additional pressure on the Emergency Department, and re-duced patient services – all of which, Nucci acknowledged, "had a demoralizing effect on everyone."

Nucci, in acting with characteristic uncompromising and straight-laced integrity, would test many of the friendships he had developed over the years. Some of his medical colleagues regarded the hospital as their personal cooperative research workshop, and they expected Nucci to support their ambition to turn St. Mary's into a mini Royal Victoria or Montreal General Hospital. Nucci had a different concept: "I liked what St. Mary's did for patients. I wanted to run a caring hos-pital, not see St. Mary's become a big-league institution for medical entrepreneurs. I couldn't allocate funds to everyone. Not all department chiefs are equal." Soon he found himself under attack from all quarters. He was held responsible for everything that went wrong at St. Mary's. Doctors had expectations of him, which, given the temper of the times, Nucci could not fulfill. In his first report as executive director, he was frank about the problems he was facing: "The increase in acute diseases of the elderly, the deinstitutionalization of psychiatric patients, has led to a significant increase in demand for medical treatment and in waiting time for patients coming to our hospital. Lack of beds for acute care patients has meant emergency corridors crowded with people waiting for admission. Various measures to relieve the congestion have been implemented, but have not been as successful as expected. Financial support from government to reopen the 30 closed beds is required."

Nucci, however, had a knack for picking bright young subordinates. When Oswald Schmidt left as his director of Finance, he brought in Larry English, who had been a supervising auditor at the Federal Business Development Bank. In spite of his name, English was a francophone from the Gaspé region. "The first thing I did was spend money to save money," he said. "I brought in computers, spent $2 million on a state-of-the-art information system, and began to put in efficiencies. I didn't believe in cutting positions. The only tools we had to work with were people, so what I did was reorganize, reinvent, and reengineer things. I had to work fast." To meet the growing need for space, the Hospital Foundation began acquiring shares in the nearby medical centre that had been built on land that the hospital had sold to a consortium of doctors in 1960, and eventually the foundation acquired the entire building.

Sean Harty left the Hospital Foundation to become Nucci's deputy. Nucci planned to groom Harty as his eventual successor. Harty was certainly qualified. While working for the hospital, he had completed an executive development program and then obtained a bachelor's degree in theology from Montreal's Concordia University. Harty had an agenda of his own, and Nucci gave him a wide berth to allow him to do whatever he thought necessary to overhaul the hospital's rehabilitative, laboratory, and educational services. Later, Harty was put in charge of all hospital services that didn't involve medicine, and he worked tirelessly to implement systems that would make the hospital run more efficiently. That did not sit well with Moralejo, who felt that his role as director of Professional Services had been denigrated. "I was prepared to be Connie's loyal lieutenant and report directly to him," Moralejo explained. "I was not prepared to report to the guy who was responsible for running the laundry and furnace rooms."

Then, in 1987, when David Schaffelburg resigned as chief of Obstetrics and Gynecology, Nucci raised eyebrows by inviting protégé Arvind Joshi, with whom he had a longstanding rapport, to take over the department. Many had taken it for granted that John Balbanian would get the job. Balbanian, an Armenian born in Egypt, had completed his degree in medicine in Cairo in 1962. He had been an intern and a resident at St. Mary's, and he had joined the staff in 1970. He was popular with both patients and staff and had spent 17 years proving himself. It seemed that the position would be his for the taking.

Joshi was East Indian, a Hindu from Nairobi, who had built a reputation specializing in high-risk obstetrics and maternal-fetal medicine. He had first come to St. Mary's as a 21-year-old extern in 1972 to spend the summer at the hospital; he was not expecting to stay. However, Nucci had liked him and decided to mentor him. Joshi went home, but two years later he returned as a landed immigrant – "with $35, a suitcase, and a medical degree" – to become a rotating intern. He finished his specialty training and learned French in Ottawa before coming to St. Mary's as an obstetrician. "I recognized someone of a different background with a superior intelligence, a young bon vivant who took medicine very seriously," Nucci recalls. "Even at his young age, I recognized a very ambitious person who was out to prove himself." Born in Uganda, Joshi was raised in Kenya, where his father ran a transport business. One of those gifted people who appear to learn effortlessly and who possess a self-assurance that can be mistaken for arrogance, Joshi turned down his father's offer to take over the family business. He had resolved to go into medicine. To support his son's ambition, Joshi's father sold his company and sent Arvind, then 17, to medical school in Dublin. There, says Joshi, "I lapped up Irish literature, theatre, and music. There was not one inch of Ireland that I didn't visit. I think of myself as more Irish than the Irish."

In 1979, within months of joining the staff at St. Mary's, Joshi realized that he didn't enjoy practising simple obstetrics and gynecology. With Nucci's encouragement, he moved to Vancouver in 1982 to take up a fellowship in high-risk pregnancies at Grace Hospital. Two years later, he moved to Regina, where he was impressed with the macro aspects of Saskatchewan healthcare. A victim of the Saskatchewan government's cuts to specialized healthcare services, Joshi was only too happy to return to Montreal, and, in January 1988, he assumed his duties at St. Mary's. Like Nucci and Quinn before him, Joshi regarded obstetrics as the heart of a community hospital: "To keep a hospital open, you only need two medical departments – obstetrics and an emergency department. By building obstetrics, you build the rest of the hospital. It is very hard to cut a hospital that has a viable obstetrics unit."

Bolstered by Nucci's confidence in him, Joshi was continuing to build and expand the department's strengths just as the deterioration in health services across the country was becoming painfully evident. As a consequence of the government's refusal to cover its operating deficits, St. Mary's was forced to reduce medical staff, close beds, and park emergency patients on gurneys in the corridors. A report to the board tells the story. It explains how in 1987, the hospital recorded a 20 percent increase in patient days, a 14 percent increase in oncology cases, a 13 percent increase in family medicine cases, a 6 percent increase in operating hours, and a 5 percent increase in emergency cases. It took 28 nurses to keep the emergency room running, but the hospital had just 17. Elective surgery was constantly being postponed, or even cancelled. In September 1988, delays in replacing the hospital's six obsolete cardiac machines restricted emergency service for several days. Patients arriving at the Emergency Department faced waits of up to five hours. Renovations had left the department with less than half its usual number of beds, and ambulance service to the hospital was cut in half. Determined to provide a secure environment for patients, Peter Duffy closed the Emergency Department in February 1989. For the first time in the history of St. Mary's, ambulances were diverted to other hospitals. "The crisis had been building," said Duffy. "The issue of emergency room crowding was kind of like a crack that was becoming more and more noticeable. We had no beds in the hospital for people who needed one. Someone was going to die. We had no choice but to close the unit and send patients to other hospitals."

There were no exceptions. A senior cardiologist on staff at St. Mary's who arrived at the Emergency Department with "troublesome symptoms" expecting preferential treatment was sent elsewhere. "The effect was disastrous for patients who needed to be admitted," said Moralejo, who objected to the closure. Nucci was hauled on the carpet by the government's regional health authority and ordered to justify the closure. "A firebrand sat there and dressed Connie down, saying he was shocked that any responsible CEO would allow his hospital to close its emergency department, describing it as a dastardly, illegal act," Duffy recalled. "Nucci stood his ground, and replied that he was shocked and amazed that the government couldn't appreciate why we had to close emergency. It was Nucci's shining hour. The whole thing turned on that meeting. Nucci stood up to the government and the government blinked."

An agreement was reached with the health ministry. In May, 24 chronic care patients who had been occupying acute care beds were moved out of St. Mary's. The Emergency Department reopened and the immediate crisis was over. Michel Tétreault, the assistant director of medical training at St. Mary's, was appointed by Quebec's health minister, Marc-Yvan Côté, to look into overcrowding in the province's emergency departments. Tétreault had been the founding president of the Quebec Association of Emergency Physicians, and since 1981 he had been advocating solutions to emergency crowding. A doctor's son, Tétreault had received his medical degree from Université de Montréal in 1975, pursued his interest in emergency medicine at McGill, and worked at the Queen Elizabeth and Lakeshore General hospitals before coming to St. Mary's in 1986. "I'd always been a loudmouth, trying to make things better," he said. "The government had spent a ton of money, and there had been no improvement in overcrowded emergencies. So, by 1989, because Dr. Nucci raised such a fuss about it, the ministry decided it needed a follow-up to the Spitzer report" – a study of seven Montreal hospitals by Claude Sicotte and Walter Spitzer, published in 1985, that examined emergency room overcrowding.

No sooner had one crisis subsided than another arose. In September, Quebec's 40,000 unionized nurses ignored essential services legislation and staged an illegal strike to back their demand for higher wages. Most of the staff nurses at St. Mary's were reluctant to join, but they were ordered off the job by their union. "The nurses at St. Mary's weren't very militant, they didn't believe in strikes, but they were pushed to the end. They had no choice," said Helene McCormack. "Any strike is demoralizing, but this one was especially so because they had no choice. The worst part was telling patients they had to go home when they weren't ready."

Through it all, management and striking nurses maintained a civil rapport. Nucci even served hot chocolate to nurses on the picket line. Ordered back to work by the government, the nurses were hit with stiff penalties and their wages were docked. Nucci had always regarded the nurses as "the backbone of the hospital," and the edict created a dilemma for him. He did not want to see the nurses penalized, but in the end he had to comply with the legislation.

CHAPTER ELEVEN

I always get into trouble with authority. I'm a renegade.
~ John Keyserlingk

Prime Minister Brian Mulroney and his wife, Mila, paid a private visit to St. Mary's in April 1990 to see their newborn nephew. Before being elected, Mulroney had been vice chairman of the hospital's $10 million fundraising campaign, and he knew the hospital well. His father-in-law, Dimitrije Pivnicki, was on the hospital's psychiatric team, and Constant Nucci had delivered Mulroney's three sons – Benedict, Mark, and Nicolas. "I loved having my babies at St. Mary's," said Mila Mulroney. "I had tough deliveries – Ben was a breach baby, and I was in labour for 24 hours with Mark. Notwithstanding the precarious nature of the deliveries, Connie Nucci was a marvellous doctor. He was divine. St. Mary's had a personal feel to it. It was around the block from where we lived. As a patient, it was as if I had all the comforts of home." Even though Mila Mulroney's father was on staff at the hospital, she was almost turned away as a patient. As Nucci tells the story, his staff hadn't realized who Mila was when she tried to book an appointment. Nucci was in the middle of a difficult delivery when Dr. Pivnicki barged into the operating theatre and demanded to know why Nucci wouldn't see his daughter.

"What's your daughter's name?" asked Nucci.

"Mulroney. Brian Mulroney's wife."

During the Prime Minister's informal visit, Nucci briefed the Mulroneys on the hospital's strategic $35 million long-range development plan: Project 2000.

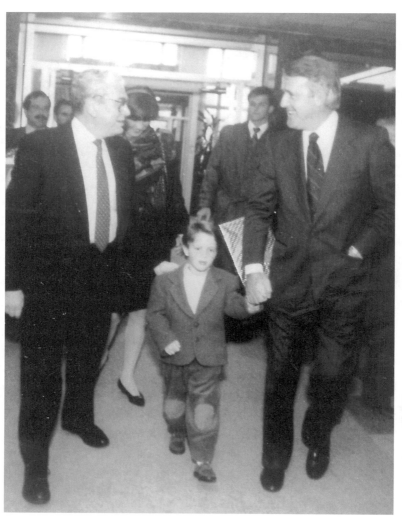

Dr. Constant Nucci greets Prime Minister Brian Mulroney, wife Mila, and son Nicolas on a visit to St. Mary's in April 1990.

The perception that St. Mary's was a faith-based institution that catered to Montreal's Irish Catholic community was no longer valid. Nucci recognized that the hospital "needed to change its image, deal with the reality, and keep pace with the changing times in medicine." If St. Mary's was to remain relevant, Nucci argued, it would have to look beyond its roots as a primary care institution and expand the secondary care it offered. To this end, Nucci proposed building on the hospital's strengths – obstetrics and family medicine – and planning ahead to provide better geriatric care for a rapidly greying population. He also proposed developing closer ties with local community health service centres (Centres locaux de services communautaires, or CLSCs) and the Father Dowd Home. Project 2000 was presented to the Quebec government in August. The timing could not have been better. A review by the Office québecois de la langue française conducted that summer found that of the 1,016 hospital employees who dealt with the public on a daily basis, 87 percent, or 880 of them, were functionally bilingual, and that there was "always someone available to provide assistance to patients in French." St. Mary's had been under increasing government pressure to keep track of employment, pension participation, and workmen's compensation data, as well as other work-related information. To satisfy the government, a computerized payroll system was introduced.

In October, Michel Tétreault, whose team had visited every hospital in the province, produced his preliminary report, which not only gave the St. Mary's emergency department high marks, but also recognized the hospital's proficiency as a patient-centred institution. Tétreault recommended a controlled SWAT-team approach to defuse critical caseloads in emergency. Because he was on staff and wished to avoid any conflict of interest, Tétreault had left it to other doctors on his team to evaluate St. Mary's. "I purposely tried to keep out of it," he said. "Before we visited a hospital, we sent out questionnaires asking the hospital to explain its policies and procedures. St. Mary's provided us with one of the shortest files of all the hospitals. It just went to prove that a hospital's capacity to actually achieve things is inversely related to what it takes to write about what it achieves."

Peter McCracken resigned as physician-in-chief to become a professor of medicine at the University of Alberta in Edmonton. Harold Zackon, a pulmonary disease specialist, succeeded him. Zackon, the son of blue-collar Jewish parents, had started at St. Mary's in the mailroom in the early 1960s while he was earning his science degree at McGill. Inspired by the dedication of an old-style family physician he knew who made house calls, Zackon went into medicine, obtaining his degree in 1971. In 1979, after training at the Royal Victoria Hospital and Hôpital Bellechasse, he accepted Guy Joron's invitation to come to St. Mary's.

There were other staff changes in 1990. John Pecknold left as chief of the Department of Psychiatry and was replaced by Martin Cole, a researcher in psychiatry and epidemiology. The hospital's surgeon-in-chief, José Rodriguez, who had been working with John Keyserlingk, was making great strides in liver resections for neoplastic disease; their techniques had attracted interest from other hospitals. But Rodriguez, increasingly frustrated by bureaucratic red tape, quit and went into private practice. "I am not an economist," he complained. "St. Mary's is a super-excellent hospital, but I was trained to be a surgeon, not spend my time being a bookkeeper for the government. More and more, I had to put up with mindless government interference when all I really wanted to do was do research and care for patients." Keyserlingk, who had recently returned from spending a leave of absence at the Royal Marsden Hospital in London, was named to replace Rodriguez. He set up a multidisciplinary head, neck, and thyroid oncology unit to diagnose and treat patients with malignant growths.

Dr. Indrojit Roy and Dr. Yasmine Ayroud established the hospital's first complete breast tumour clinic. Clinical teaching was expanded. But, like his predecessor, Keyserlingk quickly became frustrated when he realized that he had no real control over the way things were run. With disarming honesty, he remarked, "I have an intolerance for bureaucracy that gets in the way of competence. I'm competitive, and

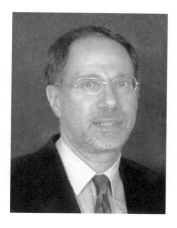

Dr. Harold Zackon succeeded Guy Joron as Physician-in-Chief.

I try to push the envelope. I was determined to have the Department of Surgery distinguish itself. I always get into trouble with authority. I'm a renegade." That attitude made Nucci increasingly uncomfortable. While Nucci appreciated Keyserlingk's enthusiasm and thought that many of his colleague's objectives were worthwhile, he had doubts about Keyserlingk's administrative ability.

Constance Lapointe stepped down as director of the Department of Family Medicine in 1991, and Mark Yaffe replaced her. To accommodate the growing number of ethical concerns related to hospital care, Dr. François Primeau, a psychogeriatrician, was hired to head a new department, which held a series of wide-ranging discussions on ethical issues such as organ transplants, living wills, and interprofessional relations. In April 1991, Quebec's labour commission – Commission des normes du travail du Québec – certified the hospital's 570 non-professional, paratechnical, and nursing care employees. In its ongoing drive to reduce the deficit, the hospital closed 27 beds on the third floor, introduced a freeze on all overtime, and began buying generic instead of brand-name drugs. It also contracted out housekeeping, laundry, meal, and maintenance services to the Marriott Corporation. The pressure of dealing with the situation created a rift among senior managers and polarized relations between Nucci and his director of

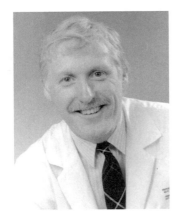

Dr. John Keyserlingk, Surgeon-in-Chief.

Professional Services, Richard Moralejo. Moralejo had been critical of a number of changes that Sean Harty was trying to implement. Nucci threw his full support behind Harty. "I have spent much time and effort trying to build a team, and I will not have it compromised by dissenting views that are not realistic nor accepted by most," he wrote to Moralejo. "I expect full support from you regarding the leadership with which both Sean and I manage this hospital." In a pointed exchange of memos, Nucci told Moralejo to resign if he could not accept Harty's management style. Ultimately, both doctors recognized that an open breach between them would have detrimental consequences for the hospital, and they agreed to "subdue" their differences. Although Nucci claimed to have "won the war," the price of that victory was a somewhat colder and much more distant relationship with his lifelong friend and colleague.

During a visit to the hospital in 1992, Quebec's health minister, Marc-Yvan Côté, pledged $2 million to St. Mary's to redesign the Emergency Department, add a trauma room, and relocate the Oncology and Ophthalmology departments. Work on remodelling the Annex began in September. With a grant from the Gustav Levinschi Foundation, the hospital was able to upgrade its nursery. To help finance the renovations, the Hospital Foundation teamed up with Hôpital Maisonneuve-Rosemont to hold the first Relais des entreprises, an annual event in which more than 300 amateur athletes representing 75 teams from the business community competed in a fundraising triathlon. Proceeds from the event were split between the two hospitals.

Revisions to the Act respecting Health Services and Social Services in the autumn of 1992 created three new entities – the council of physicians, dentists and pharmacists, the multidisciplinary council and the council of nurses – and put St. Mary's into a new category: university-affiliated hospitals. St. Mary's was also brought into the regional administrative health unit, and this meant that changes had to be made to the makeup of its board. New regulations required representation from the university and from medical staff. Arvind Joshi, who had recently completed his MBA at Concordia University's John Molson School of Business, was elected representative of the hospital's Council of Physicians, Dentists, and Pharmacists to the Board of Directors. The legislation also demanded modifications to the hospital's strategic long-range development plan.

The hospital's reputation as a birthing centre was enhanced in April 1993, when Joshi delivered the first set of quintuplets to be born in Quebec by Caesarean section. Joshi was part of a high-risk team led by Apostolos Papageorgiou, chief of Pediatrics and Neonatology at the Jewish General Hospital. The story made headlines around the world, and Joshi's name figured prominently. But not all news coverage that year related to St. Mary's was laudatory. At the end of 1992, St. Mary's was shaken by negative publicity when investigators with the U.S. National Cancer Institute and the Office of Research Integrity, as part of the National Surgical Adjuvant Breast and Bowel Project, monitored the hospital's tamoxifen research program and announced that they suspected doctors of fabricating evidence. Shaken by the "extremely serious" allegations, the Collège des médecins du Québec conducted its own impartial investigation and concluded that clerical errors were made during an audit and there was no substance to the allegations. Keyserlingk's secretary accepted responsibility for the mistake. The incident further strained relations between Keyserlingk and Nucci, as Nucci was now convinced that administrative chaos reigned in Keyserlingk's department.

"As brilliant as he is, when it came to paperwork, [Keyserlingk] was careless. But that's not a firing offense," said Nucci. Then Nucci discovered that Keyserlingk had booked operating suites for elective surgery three months in advance during a period in July that was reserved for emergency cases. Anticipating his department's requirements, Keyserlingk had reserved these suites in the names of fictitious patients to keep them available should they be needed. That, in Nucci's mind, *was* a firing offense. "This was a big deal for me," Nucci explained. "I could appreciate him wanting to reserve space for his doctors in advance, but ethically, given what we had just gone through with the Office of Integrity, this was not the way to do it." Nucci demanded Keyserlingk's resignation. Supported by Center Board chairman Norman Byrne, Nucci asked Dr. Carl Émond, a vascular surgeon who had been a past director of surgical teaching, to fill in until a replacement could be found. At first, Keyserlingk agreed to resign, then he changed his mind. The impasse led to a rift among the various department heads; they chose their sides in the dispute. Some colleagues, most notably Moralejo – who had already announced that he was stepping down after 20 years as director of Professional Services – did not want to see Keyserlingk fired. Moralejo agreed that falsifying documents using names of nonexistent patients was a major offense. "I was ready to strangle Keyserlingk, and I knew he had to be reprimanded. But Connie overruled me and said he was going to deal with it his way. He asked me to stay out of it. I thought Connie had crossed a line by interfering and going over my head. But I did. I stayed out of it."

In March 1993, with Keyserlingk still refusing to quit, Nucci decided to lodge a formal complaint against him with the hospital's Council of Physicians, Dentists, and Pharmacists. As far as Nucci was con-

cerned, the issue was one of "integrity, honesty, leadership, and trust."
By then, Hugh Whalen, a paper company executive, had been made
chairman of the Center Board. Whalen pointed out that Keyserlingk's
appointment as surgeon-in-chief would expire in 1996. He proposed
that Keyserlingk be allowed to finish his term with the understanding
that his appointment would not be renewed. Nucci wanted none of it.
He refused to postpone the dismissal, which he thought should be
effective immediately. "Once the ball got rolling and I got involved, I
did not think it was reasonable to give Keyserlingk more time," Nucci
explained. A committee set up to deal with the situation repeatedly
stalled, and the matter simmered.

All the while, St. Mary's kept building its relationship with McGill.
The university moved its Centre for Studies in Aging to St. Mary's in
July 1993. Under the direction of Serge Gauthier, the centre concentrated on clinical research in the field of gerontology. The Department of Clinical Epidemiology and Community Studies, headed by
Jane McCusker, also opened in 1993, signalling a departure from
bench research. As well, half the family medicine residents training
at the Montreal General were transferred to St. Mary's. Two divisions
were added to the Department of Family Medicine: in-hospital family physicians and community family physicians. "There were still
some people around who felt we shouldn't bother with McGill because the university got more from us than we received from it," said
Nucci. "But I recognized that even if we were shortchanged and didn't
get the financial compensation we deserved for the work we were
doing for McGill, we had to accept it. In the long run, it was worth it
for patient care."

That summer, St. Mary's also held its first annual golf tournament
at the Summerlea Golf and Country Club, raising $50,000 for an
anesthesia machine to be used in the operating rooms. With the renovations to the powerhouse complete, Gerald Berry at last moved into
his long-awaited autopsy suite, which had four times as much space
as the old one. The suite was later used for a scene in Jean Beaudin's
2002 film *Le collectionneur*, starring Luc Picard.

In the autumn of 1994, St. Mary's became a campus for the University of Ottawa's bachelor of science in nursing program; three years later, it would produce its first graduate. Sean Harty, who had completed his studies for the priesthood, was ordained on October 1, 1993. Although he was named curate of St. Veronica's Parish in Dorval, Harty continued to serve as the hospital's associate executive director. He supported the traditional approach of the Catholic Church, "where priests are presidents of universities, where the religious run hospitals and large conglomerates," and he believed that he could do both jobs. His stress level increased when the Quebec government imposed staff cuts of 20 percent and ordered the laboratory to cut costs by 10 percent. Harty assured the board that "while the process will be complex and painful, every effort will be made to minimize the impact on our personnel." To his credit, Harty kept the ministry informed of what was going on at St. Mary's, bombarding bureaucrats with balance sheets so they could not ignore the hospital's efficiency – a strategy that would pay off in the long run.

Marvin Kwitko was appointed chief of the Department of Ophthalmology in the autumn of 1994. Kwitko was also associate professor of ophthalmology at McGill, where he taught the only course of its kind in Canada on laser surgery; he would train more than 350 surgeons. He also advised Health Canada on excimer laser surgery. The author of five textbooks, Kwitko had hoped to write even more, but he died in 2002.

The internal administrative debacle over Keyserlingk's authority, or lack of it, persisted in slow motion. As Nucci grappled with the problem, his singlemindedness undermined morale, and it eventually cost him the support of many staff doctors, who believed that he had betrayed their interests. On March 21, 1994, the doctors met to address the issue. Based on a 100-to-6 vote, they decided to censure Nucci. The following Thursday, a delegation in support of Keyserlingk – which included executive members of the Council of Physicians, Dentists, and Pharmacists – appeared before the Center Board. Nucci came pre-

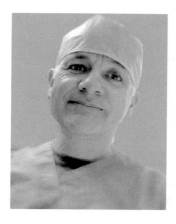

Dr. Carl Émond stepped in
as Surgeon-in-Chief.

pared for the showdown. If the board refused to fire Keyserlingk, then he, Nucci, was going to quit. During the meeting, Nucci was challenged by two doctors (their names are not recorded in the board minutes), who insisted, "You have indicated that Keyserlingk had committed a major infraction, yet for all other bodies this constitutes a minor infraction." The board then met *in camera* to consider Nucci's resolution: "Whereas J.R. Keyserlingk has failed to show leadership and the exemplary behaviour that [befits] his position as Surgeon-in-Chief, it is in the interests of this hospital that his contract be terminated." Forced to choose between the hospital's CEO and a department head, the Center Board not only voted to support Nucci, but it also went on record as commending him for his "diligence" and the "proper manner in which he attempted to ensure the highest standards of behaviour at all times by all levels of staff."

With that, Carl Émond was confirmed as chief of surgery. Émond, born in Ottawa, grew up in St-Jean-sur-Richelieu, where his father was in the Canadian Air Force. After obtaining an arts degree from Université de Montréal in 1970, he went into medicine, and he completed his degree at McGill University seven years later. In 1985, he initiated a vascular clinic at St. Mary's and established the hospital's vascular lab. He was reluctant to take over as surgeon-in-chief "because of the disarray in the healthcare system, and because of the hard decisions I knew I would have to make."

The manner in which Keyserlingk was dismissed had infuriated many on staff. Through Arvind Joshi, who was its representative on the Center Board, the Council of Physicians, Dentists, and Pharmacists asked the board to reconsider its decision. Joshi had to straddle the fence and be both physician and manager as he spoke of the "negative mood of animosity" that was lingering in the aftermath of the affair. As both department chief and board member, Joshi was between a rock and a hard place. Having the capacity to compartmentalize his various duties, he was able to consider the legal angles. Finally, he felt satisfied that "due process" had been followed in the Keyserlingk affair. The matter was closed.

The issue now behind him, Nucci turned to much more serious concerns. The federal government was running a deficit equal to one-quarter of its annual budget – nearly 6 percent of the gross national product. It responded by reducing health transfer payments to the provinces. This, in turn, increased the pressure the Quebec government was exerting on the hospitals, and so St. Mary's had to cut staff. To answer the ministry's demand that it cut lab costs, the hospital also reorganized its cytology laboratory. Then St. Mary's decided to farm out its Pap tests (for cervical cancer) on a six-month trial basis to Excel Bestview, a private laboratory in Mississauga, Ontario, that used state-of-the-art laser technology unavailable in Quebec. When she found out about this, the Quebec health minister, Lucienne Robillard, reprimanded Nucci for what she called his "inexplicable and unacceptable" decision to deal with an Ontario lab without permission from the Regional Health Board. St. Mary's cancelled the arrangement. "An election had been called. The government didn't want to be embarrassed by a political uproar that might be caused if the opposition found out that tests that should have been done in Quebec were being done in Ontario," said Nucci. "It didn't cost anybody anything, and might have even saved us money. It was a comparative study. Excel Bestview was going to do our Pap tests, and we were going to do its prostate tests [PSAs]. It was an unbelievably traumatic time for me."

Subjected to such convulsions in the healthcare system, St. Mary's not only slashed its laboratory staff, but also lost 45 full-time doctors and nurses, as well as 19 part-time employees, who took buyouts. Despite the constraints, and despite everything St. Mary's had endured that year, the Canadian Council on Health Services Accreditation had high praise "for the quality of services offered to patients" at St. Mary's and for the "warm, caring environment [that] prevails."

As Physician-in-Chief, Harold Zackon had to contend with the sharp reduction in house staff. McGill stopped sending residents to St. Mary's, and it became extremely difficult to recruit qualified people. "We had only specialists left, so, out of necessity, we developed a model at St. Mary's that paired a specialist with a family physician," Zackon explained. Dr. George Michaels was the first specialist to be hired to mentor a family physician, and he was put in charge of the new in-hospital family physicians division. "Gradually," said Zackon, "all patients were put under the day-to-day care of rotating family physicians who were responsible for the primary care of patients who had been admitted by a specialist." There was an explosion in the number of specialists and subspecialists. Ron Onerheim, the hospital's new chief pathologist, was one standout among the new recruits. That year, he won the coveted Osler Award for Outstanding Teaching. Originally from Regina, Saskatchewan, Onerheim graduated from the University of Alberta at the top of his class in 1978 and came to Montreal the following year to study at McGill.

In May, Arvind Joshi, who had just been certified by the Canadian College of Health Executives, took over from Moralejo as director of Professional Services. Dr. Normand Brassard replaced Joshi as head of Obstetrics and Gynecology. Brassard, today professor and chair of obstetrics and gynecology at Université Laval, would be instrumental in setting up a comprehensive obstetrical database and helping the hospital's program manager design the new $2.6 million birthing

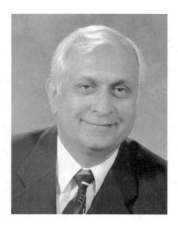

Dr. Arvind K. Joshi.

centre. From this fresh vantage point, Joshi was well positioned to
assess the strengths and weaknesses of the hospital staff. He pondered
strategies for improving how the hospital was run, considered new and
different ways it could function, and thought about its relationship
to government. He also acknowledged the existence of a certain
underlying tension between the religious and secular natures of the
institution. Joshi's ascendency was resented in certain quarters, not
because he was East Indian, but because he was regarded by some as a
brash and ambitious technocrat and a sycophant who had thrown his
unconditional support behind Nucci during the Keyserlingk affair.
"Everybody knew I was 'Nucci's boy,'" he said. "But what none of our
critics appreciated was no matter how close we are, we are both exceptionally professional." Joshi was suave, decisive, and confident, and he
had a mind of his own; some thought his demeanour was out of step
with the hospital's traditional close-knit corporate culture. One board
member remarked, "Joshi listened a lot, observed a lot, rarely spoke,
but you could always hear the wheels turning inside his head."

In the spring of 1995, Nucci created the position of chief operating officer, and Sean Harty, still climbing the corporate ladder, was put
in charge of the hospital's day-to-day operations. A clinical advisory
committee was established to permit the chiefs of all the medical

departments a greater say in administration. However, while such changes were introduced to compensate for staff shortages and to encourage greater individual participation in the running of St. Mary's, they actually blurred the lines of authority. Senior managers began to question each other's motives and be suspicious of one another.

Then, on May 11, 1995, without any warning or explanation, the Quebec government closed eight Montreal community hospitals: the Queen Elizabeth, Lachine General, Reddy Memorial, St-Laurent, Ste-Jeanne-d'Arc, Bellechasse, Guy Laporte, and Gouin-Rosemont. Much soul-searching has gone on since that time in an attempt to understand why the Queen Elizabeth, one of the city's oldest English-language community hospitals, once as good as St. Mary's and certainly better situated, was targeted and St. Mary's was spared. The Queen Elizabeth was founded in 1895 as the Homeopathic Hospital of Montreal, and it had in some ways been coasting on its century-old reputation. It had also suffered severe management problems – going through four CEOs in six years – and it had been at a distinct disadvantage since 1973, when its obstetrics department had closed. In a nutshell, Nucci and Harty had learned how to massage the government, and they had done the government's bidding. The Queen Elizabeth had not. By the time it hired its first francophone director general – Mario Larivière, in 1993 – it was already too late.

The closing of the Queen Elizabeth was, in many respects, the salvation of St. Mary's. The Queen Elizabeth's palliative care and oncology services were integrated into those of St. Mary's, and 63 Queen Elizabeth employees were redeployed to St. Mary's. Room was made for three Queen Elizabeth orthopedic surgeons – Larry Lincoln, Larry Coughlin, and Joyce Johansson – and this enhanced the sports medicine division. The St. Mary's Hospital Foundation received one-third of the Queen Elizabeth Hospital Foundation's money: $2 million. St. Mary's also got the Queen Elizabeth's CT scan machine and all of its medical records. Élisabeth Dampolias, coordinator of Patient Information Services at St. Mary's, negotiated with Montreal's Régie régionale de la santé to scan all 600,000 medical records from both the Queen Elizabeth and the Reddy Memorial to assure continuity of patient care.

The government's abrupt hospital closures, which took 1,000 beds out of circulation, were as unnerving as they were disruptive. The immediate impact on St. Mary's was a 30 percent increase in emergency patients and a 20 percent increase in oncology patients; and the number of chronic care patients rose from an average of 50 to an average of 100. After balancing its budget for two years, St. Mary's now faced a $3.5 million deficit.

"We were surrounded by three giant hospitals – the Jewish General, the Montreal General, and the Royal Victoria – all 10 minutes away from us. We were worried," admitted Zackon. "It was difficult to predict what the government's next action would be." It was the summer of a second referendum on Quebec's future. The campaign was waged for several months, and the political uncertainty was demoralizing. In Ottawa, Paul Martin, the federal finance minister, vowed that "come hell or high water," he would put the country back on a sound financial footing, even if it meant slashing healthcare. It looked as if Quebec separatists might win their referendum. In June, to deal with the rising level of anxiety, Harty convened a retreat of 80 managers at the Estérel Resort and Convention Centre, located north of Montreal on a Laurentian lake. Out of the brainstorming session came an interdisciplinary approach to hospital management that would involve a continued organizational learning team (COLT). Harty's idea was to promote team-building skills and to "coach all employees in various departments throughout the hospital so they would have a greater appreciation of each other's jobs and all become interdependent and more responsible caregivers."

The Quebec government continued to restructure healthcare services. In April, it announced the voluntary merger of five English-speaking hospitals – the Royal Victoria Hospital, the Montreal General Hospital, the Montreal Children's Hospital, the Montreal Neurological Institute and Hospital, and the Montreal Chest Institute – into one acute care hospital and research centre, which was to be called the McGill Academic Health Sciences Centre.

The government established several categories of hospitals in Quebec: centres hospitaliers universitaires, or CHUs (affiliated with the four medical schools in Quebec and Ste-Justine was also designated a CHU, for a total of five in the province); the other designations were called centres hospitaliers affiliés universitaires, or CHAUs; and single specialty institutes like the Montreal Heart Institute. St. Mary's did not receive an official designation but retained its close relationship with McGill. McGill's dean of medicine, Richard Cruess, supported St. Mary's claim that it should be assigned to the CHAU category. There was widespread concern that the government was about to close St. Mary's. "St. Mary's will have to work to reposition its focus if it expects to have a future," Nucci warned. However, the government's go-between, Marcel Villeneuve, head of the Régie régionale, assured Nucci that the government would never close St. Mary's because it considered the hospital a "model for all other hospitals in the province."

St. Mary's may have been a model, but, as director of Professional Services, Arvind Joshi came to appreciate the need to decentralize its management: "We began talking about looking beyond the traditional management organization and looking at a more patient-friendly system of program management. We wanted to see what worked and what didn't work." Ralph Dadoun, who reported to Joshi, had visited the Markham Stouffville Hospital, an acute care and general community facility in Markham, Ontario; and he had also toured St. Joseph's Hospital in Toronto. Both had gone from department-based to program-based management and seen significant savings. Joshi became convinced that St. Mary's could do the same.

In addition to being head of Professional Services, Joshi became, in September, head of the joint Jewish General–St. Mary's Division of Perinatal Medicine. Between the two hospitals, 8,000 babies were being delivered each year, so the appointment made sense administratively. Renovations to the fourth-floor birthing centre were started

– larger rooms were created to accommodate 40 postpartum beds, with a crib and a chair-bed for the father in each room. A drive-through garage for ambulances was added, and $2.6 million was spent on renovations to the sixth-floor nursing station and to emergency facilities; a new health sciences library was also built. Dadoun again restructured the Department of Laboratories, introducing the first self-sufficient core lab in Quebec. "Not only did we cut costs, we maintained the lab's quality and high standards, increased the efficiency of portable tests, decreased the physical lab space, and reduced staff by 16 percent," he pointed out. As a result, the lab was accredited by the program of excellence of the College of American Pathologists; it was the only laboratory in Quebec, and one of three in Canada, to be recognized as having the highest standards on the continent.

In October, the hospital foundation embarked on a $14 million capital fundraising campaign, which, appropriately, was launched at Shaughnessy House, where St. Mary's Hospital began in 1924. As part of a program advertised as "A New Era of Family Care," Nucci promoted a policy of closer cooperation with other hospitals. Balancing the sometimes contradictory demands of the government with what he thought was best for St. Mary's, and constantly working on a cost-quality analysis, fatigued Nucci. St. Mary's was expected to keep up with the latest advances in medical technology, even as operating budgets were being slashed. The Keyserlingk affair had made Nucci feel isolated and disconnected from his subordinates. With the death in February 1996 of former board chairman Norman Byrne, he found himself without a loyal and trusted ally at the Center Board level. He was losing the heart he needed to run the hospital.

It all came to a head on Wednesday, May 22, 1996. There was an especially stressful combined meeting of the Center Board and senior management. Nucci had no intention of quitting that day, but as the meeting progressed and various presentations were made, he felt he "had lost the ball. I felt I was being undermined at every turn." When the meeting broke for lunch, Nucci made up his mind to throw in the

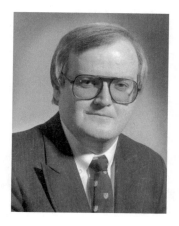

Sean Harty, a Roman Catholic priest, became acting CEO in 1996.

towel. "There is a time to come and a time to go, and the time has come for me to go," he told the astonished Center Board chairman, Hugh Whalen, as he handed in his resignation. He was leaving, he said, "with a sense of nostalgia for the good old days, and grief for the times in which we live."

Nucci was asked to join the hospital's board of governors, but, "for personal reasons relating to my values, strong views on leadership, and the handling of contentious issues," he decided to make a clean break with the hospital that had been his life for four decades. "I must decline," he told Whalen. "I feel this is in the best interests of the institution at this time." The hospital was thrown into confusion by the unexpected resignation. Sean Harty moved into Nucci's office as interim CEO, fully expecting the search committee to confirm his appointment as CEO. "Under the circumstances, Harty's appointment was a natural progression," said Whalen. "There were people around who thought we should forget our roots as a Catholic institution, and we as a board were not prepared to do that." Harty was eager to assert his leadership, but because of the significant divisions at both board and management levels over how to manage the growing hospital and its deficit, he was unsure of his footing.

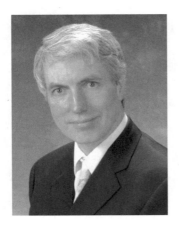

Dr. Todd McConnell, Physician-in-Chief.

While some board members voiced their concern that the hospital had drifted away from its Irish Catholic roots, the Irish Catholic community could no longer be counted upon for its financial support. "The tensions within the administration were at many levels," Harty said. "All of the departments were in transition. We had to look at whether the management structures that we had were making the place better, or whether they were obstructing progress. There were some difficult moments, because many people thought that change meant destroying the very essence of a Catholic hospital."

In truth, St. Mary's had not been a Catholic hospital for years, although there were still some who refused to accept it. By 1996, only one in five patients identified as Roman Catholic. The St. Mary's brand name no longer meant very much to the majority of patients and staff. Todd McConnell, who became Physician-in-Chief when Harold Zackon relinquished the post in 1996, illustrated the point with a telling anecdote. McConnell had arrived at St. Mary's sporting a beard. "We had a lot of long-term care patients, and it was not unusual as you were walking down the hall to hear people call out 'Doctor, Doctor.' I used to get 'Doctor, Doctor' a fair bit. But I guess my beard got to a certain length, and one day I was walking down the hall when suddenly I heard, 'Rabbi, Rabbi.'" In fact, by then the hospital counted almost as many Jews among its patients as it did Catholics.

A specialist in internal medicine, McConnell was born in Minneapolis, Minnesota. He studied at Carleton College in Northfield, Minnesota, and he went on to Wisconsin Medical College for his medical degree. In 1973, he landed at the Royal Victoria Hospital. He then spent a year at an Antarctica research station before obtaining his license to practise medicine in Quebec in 1979. In 1988, McConnell was lecturing at McGill and serving as director of Ambulatory Care at the Royal Victoria when Peter McCracken invited him to come to St. Mary's as an attending physician.

While McConnell settled in as physician-in-chief, Harty was left to grapple with the hospital's unprecedented $4 million deficit. In addition to his priestly commitments, he now had to cope with the influx of new patients, the staff arriving from other institutions due to hospital closures, and the brain drain caused by the government buyouts offered to its doctors and nurses. To further complicate matters, the province's healthcare deficit was approaching $250 million, and the Montreal region accounted for half of that. Faced with dire budget cuts, Quebec's health minister, Jean Rochon, admitted that the health system was on the brink of collapse, and he closed even more ERs. Urgences-santé, the province's ambulance service, complained that it could no longer function because so many ERs had closed. The Régie régionale chopped another 52 positions at St. Mary's, including 33 nursing positions. Harty was alarmed by the brain drain. In order to streamline patient services, the hospital opened a walk-in clinic on September 1, 1996.

When the selection committee to choose Nucci's permanent replacement was named, Alain Benedetti, a no-nonsense chartered accountant and a member of the Center Board, was put in charge. Italian-born Benedetti had been involved in fundraising and was all too aware of the hospital's ingrained inefficiencies. "There had been issues," he said diplomatically. "I was surprised at what had been taking place, and I voiced my displeasure at board meetings. It was obvious we needed change. A break with the past. We needed totally new management."

In order to build a consensus, Benedetti began soliciting professional outside advice on how St. Mary's should be run. As the year dragged on, Harty was made aware that Joshi was being consulted about a radical overhaul of the hospital administration based on the Markham Stouffville model, and that his advice was being taken seriously at the board level. Satisfied "that an outsider would probably not be brought in to run St. Mary's," Harty resigned, with certain misgivings, accepting a position at Concordia University as a full-time professor in the theology department. He postponed leaving his position as acting director until October 23, 1997, when the selection committee announced Joshi's appointment.

Summing up his 15-year career at the hospital, Harty said that the moment he first arrived at St. Mary's, he had fallen for the people who worked there, adding, "I am still under their spell, and always will be. Even though all of us did not agree on how to solve particular problems, we all shared a deep, common understanding of patient-focused care." In 2002, Harty was appointed episcopal vicar of Montreal's English-speaking Roman Catholic community, a position he held until 2011.

CHAPTER TWELVE

Things at St. Mary's were in disarray. The hospital was not just facing winds of change but a tsunami of change. Once again, St. Mary's had to face its future.
~ Arvind Joshi

৵

Arvind Joshi's appointment as chief executive officer put an end to a generally demoralizing chapter in the hospital's evolution. With swift bureaucratic efficiency, Joshi helped St. Mary's to usher in a new era. There would be dramatic changes to the way the hospital was administered. Joshi was "decisive, he knew what he wanted, and he knew where he was going," said one of his subordinates. "Not only could he see the big picture, he could see three frames ahead."

A lean new management team was introduced to oversee the transformation of St. Mary's from a department-based institution into a program-management-based hospital. The management team hit the ground running in the first week of January 1998, just as Montreal was paralyzed by an ice storm that left it without electricity for the better part of a week. During the catastrophe, the hospital's Emergency Department outperformed all others on the Island of Montreal. St. Mary's handled more than 800 patients. Most were treated within 12 hours, and only a few had to be hospitalized for more than a couple of days. As the crisis intensified, the hospital provided temporary shelter to 900 people. Volunteers assisted in the preparation and service of more than 2,000 meals. St. Mary's also offered daycare services during the storm's aftermath. For its efforts, St. Mary's was rewarded with a $200,000 incentive bonus from the government.

"There was a period of adjustment," says Todd McConnell. "We had been used to working with a variety of people and reporting to a single program manager. But ultimately, structure isn't nearly as

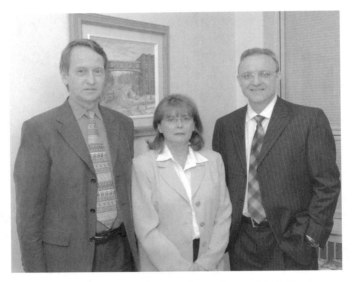

A new management team takes over: Bruce Brown, Linda Bambonye, and Ralph Dadoun.

important as the patients you're treating. The bottom line is, if you hire a great program manager, you get a great program. If you hire a poor manager, you are going to have a poor program. It is the people in charge who carry the day for you." Those who had been brought in to carry the day included Ralph Dadoun, who was installed as vice president of Corporate Support Services, which had absorbed what was the Financial Services Department. Larry English had conveniently resigned as director of Financial Services just before the new management team took over to accept a similar job at Concordia University.

The director of the Department of Nursing, Helene McCormack, took the government buyout package. Her title was retired, and Linda Bambonye, who had come to St. Mary's from the Montreal General, was named vice president for Operations and Nursing. Bambonye, who had trained as a biologist, was a graduate of Montreal's Marianopolis College. She had worked as a lab technician before leaving for Burundi to teach biology. While there, she recognized that a nursing degree would be useful to her if she wanted to continue to work in Africa. She returned home to obtain her degree from Université de Montréal, but she never went back to Africa. At St. Mary's, she would be responsible not only for the nursing staff but also for all rehabilitation services, respiratory therapy services, and social services. The admitting office and the Medical Records Department would also come under her jurisdiction. A whole new crew was attached to the nursing department, and it would take Bambonye about two-and-a-half years to produce all the necessary job descriptions and to get things running smoothly. Nurses went from being completely in charge of their patients to being part of a system that involved multiple healthcare professionals, including physiotherapists and occupational therapists. A structure was set up to facilitate the professional development of all of the allied health professionals.

Dr. Bruce Brown – who held degrees from McGill, Johns Hopkins, and McMaster Universities, and who had been with the Department of Family Medicine since 1976 – was named vice president of Professional Services in February. The hospital's dental clinic was closed, and the CT scan machine that St. Mary's had inherited from the Queen Elizabeth Hospital was installed. The hospital's information system was upgraded. A method of front-loading patients to save money in the operating rooms was introduced. Surgeries that required patients to be hospitalized for three or four days were scheduled early in the week, and surgeries requiring shorter stays were booked at the end of the week, which allowed the hospital to economize by closing beds on weekends.

St. Mary's had emerged from its trials in a state of internal coherence that set it apart from the city's other hospitals. Having reformed the administrative structure, Joshi and his team embarked on a thorough, far-reaching review of St. Mary's relationship with McGill University. Although St. Mary's continued to fulfill its contractual obligations to the university by training residents in the Department of

Family Medicine, the hospital's wider role within the healthcare system had still not been clearly defined. Dr. Abraham Fuks, dean of McGill University Faculty of Medicine, agreed that from a training and service perspective, St. Mary's was indispensible to McGill.

Another radical break with the past was the appointment, in 1998, of Richard Renaud to the board of the St. Mary's Hospital Foundation. A chartered accountant with a dynamic personality, Renaud was a founding partner of private investment firm Wynnchurch Capital. A "Loyola boy," Renaud had agreed to help St. Mary's because, "in the world I live in, that's what was expected of someone who was educated by Jesuits." Renaud was a merchant banker who possessed the expertise to reduce financial and economic complexities to a common-sense level. He had made his fortune by buying and reinvigorating failing businesses, then selling them at a profit. A hands-on philanthropist, he operated below the radar out of a Place Ville Marie office filled with Canadian art. He served as vice chair of Concordia University's board of directors and its foundation. At Concordia, he had helped to reengineer the institution by chopping $45 million from its operating budget. He then raised the money to build the John Molson School of Business and the science centre that bears his name. Renaud turned down an offer to join the board of the Montreal General Hospital because he thought he could "do more for, and make things happen at St. Mary's."

Renaud quickly immersed himself in the daily life of St. Mary's and started tapping into new sources of revenue for the foundation. He created an endowment fund to refurbish the Family Medicine Centre in the old nurses' residence and increased the foundation's fundraising targets by 25 percent each year. He also stepped on a few toes when he assumed direct responsibility for the St. Mary's Ball, which for 60 years had been the exclusive preserve of the Ladies Auxiliary. With Renaud in charge, the 1998 ball raised $250,000 – twice as much as the auxiliary-mounted affair the previous year. "It was a party with a renewed spirit, with the theme of 'For the Love of St. Mary's,'" reported the gossip columnist for the *Gazette*. "More than 400 people

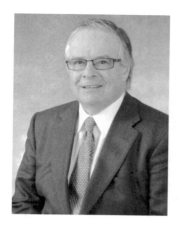

Rick Renaud, philanthropist.

turned out and partied like mad....What really rejuvenated the ball was that a lot of new people came to support St. Mary's." Renaud also acted to raise the Hospital Foundation's profile. He engaged Cynda P. Heward, director of development at the Montreal General, as the foundation's first president and chief operating officer. The daughter of a Vancouver entrepreneur, Heward obtained a degree in economics from Queen's University and worked as a money-market manager at Wood Gundy before earning her stripes as a fundraiser for British Colombia Children's Hospital. St. Mary's was not on her radar screen. When Renaud offered her the job, she wasn't sure where the hospital was. She was won over on her first visit. As she put it, "I likened St. Mary's to the atmosphere at Cheers...it was a place where everybody knew your name. It was community-oriented, a place where people could make a difference. I was ready to do more, so I accepted the challenge."

There were more revitalizing changes in store. In 1999, when Alain Benedetti's term as Center Board chairman ended, he recommended a total outsider, Dr. Sarah Prichard, as his replacement. Prichard had no ties to St. Mary's and was virtually an unknown to the board members. Her nomination represented the final break with the "old Irish gentlemen's club" that had run the hospital since its founding. She was the first woman to head the board and the first physician to take the reins since the hospital's founding chairman, Donald Hingston, took them in 1924. Prichard arrived wearing two hats: that of board chair; and that of associate dean of Inter-hospital Affairs at McGill, where she had helped write the rules and set the specifications for hospitals affiliated with the university. Not since Guy Joron had St. Mary's employed someone so capable of appreciating the mutual interests of hospital and university. The daughter of a British physician, Prichard was born in Boston, grew up in Toronto, and studied medicine at Queen's University, where she was awarded her degree in 1974. She built her career in the Department of Medicine at the Royal Victoria, where she was chief of service and director of the peritoneal dialysis unit. She taught at McGill, and in 1992 she received the Osler Award. "If St. Mary's really intended to be serious about spreading its wings, it had to become more proactive and a little less folksy and laid-back," Prichard commented. "The biggest challenge was to up the ante and recruit a much more dynamic board – people who were not necessarily sentimentally, historically, or culturally attached to St. Mary's. Some people were asked to retire from the board to make way for new blood. Because I was an outsider, it is perhaps something only I could have done." Prichard worked with Renaud and Joshi to develop a strategy that, "from the start, was to apply to the government to have St. Mary's designated a university-affiliated hospital. My appointment was all about cementing St. Mary's to McGill and getting the government to designate the hospital as an autonomous teaching hospital. St. Mary's was already training 12 percent of the students from the McGill Faculty of Medicine."

St. Mary's celebrated its 75th anniversary in 1999 with a ball that took as its theme the Roaring Twenties. More than $360,000 was raised for the Family Medicine Centre. The foundation was able to buy a gamma camera to use in nuclear medicine, as well as new dialysis, echocardiographic, urological, and endoscopic equipment. A made-for-television movie, *One Special Night*, starring Julie Andrews and James Garner, was shot on location at the hospital that year. Andrews

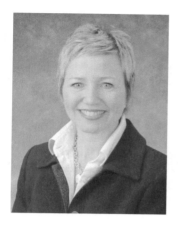

Cynda P. Heward, president and CEO of
the St. Mary's Hospital Foundation.

played a widowed pediatrician who keeps returning to the room in
which her husband died. She especially enjoyed the film shoot, and
she commented on how friendly, without being deferential, the hospital staff had been to her.

The Canadian Council on Health Services Accreditation (CCHSA),
which examined the hospital that autumn, commended the new
senior management team and the Center Board for their effective
leadership. "Clinical guidelines and performance indicators are more
extensively used, and links with the community and McGill University have been strengthened," the CCHSA reported. "Community
groups now have better access to the hospital's facilities, there is an
active volunteer group, and many hospital personnel are involved in
external agencies."

To mark the arrival of the millennium in 2000, an anonymous
donor equipped the hospital with a full-service gymnasium that
boasted state-of-the-art cardiovascular and bodybuilding machines
for the exclusive use of the staff. February 1 saw the opening of a
medical day centre, designed to relieve congestion in the Emergency
Department. With an emphasis on ambulatory care, the centre handled 5,000 patients annually. Some of them, who might otherwise

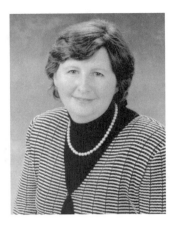

Dr. Sarah Prichard, first woman
to become hospital board chair.

have been admitted, were able to recover in their own homes. Six spots
in the centre were reserved for patients arriving at the Emergency
Department. "In the future, only the very sick are going to be hospitalized," said the head nurse, Sylvie Larocque. "We have a 90 percent
success rate; only 10 percent of the patients we admit require surgery.
Most of our patients go home, sleep in their own beds, go to work,
shop, and remain with their families while they are being treated."

In April, the Hospital Foundation initiated a fundraising program
to refurbish the family medicine and birthing centres. In order to
supervise the project, Richard Renaud became head of the Center
Board; his sister, Rachel, eventually became foundation board president. Amendments to the bill governing health services required the
Center Board to reduce its membership from 21 to 17 and to include
two new representatives: one from the regional health services centre,
and one from another institution. To better serve the community,
the hospital launched a website (www.smhc.qc.ca). While it was intent
on discarding those things that were no longer relevant at St. Mary's,
the board was careful to uphold traditions that were still meaningful
to many of its supporters. Abortions, for example, have never been
performed at the hospital, even though it is no longer a Roman
Catholic institution. A memorial plot for stillborn and miscarried

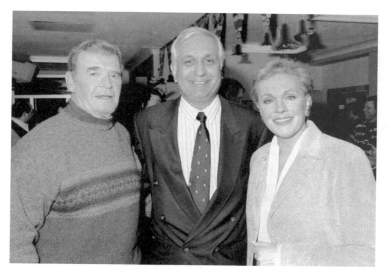

James Garner, Arvind Joshi, and Julie Andrews on the set of the movie *One Special Night* shot at St. Mary's.

infants was acquired; a stone marker was installed there bearing the hospital logo and the inscription "Nos Tout-petits, Jamais Oubliés, Pour Toujours dans nos Coeurs" ("Our little ones, Never forgotten, Forever in our hearts").

When John Sutton, who had been director of Orthopedics for 12 years, took over as chief of surgery from Carl Émond in 2003, he became the first non-general surgeon to fill the position. Sutton's father had been a surgeon at the Montreal General for half a century; his older brother, Carl, was also an orthopedic surgeon. Known around the hospital as "Big Jack," Sutton was a Loyola graduate who had excelled in football, baseball, and squash; he earned his medical degree at McGill.

Rick Renaud remained as board chair until 2009, but those who followed him – Marc Trottier and James Cherry – have similar clout in the community. Trottier, who served until 2012, was a senior partner at, and director of Jarislowsky Fraser Investment, and Cherry, the current board chair, is also president and chief executive officer of Aéroports de Montréal.

St. Mary's was pushed into a new league when the board applied to the Quebec government in 2003 to have the institution designated a university-affiliated hospital centre. Given the government's warm relationship with McGill, it was anticipated that the upgrade would be almost automatic. But when it comes to healthcare, nothing in the bureaucratic world is ever routine. Each time a government changes – be it in Ottawa or in Quebec City – the healthcare industry holds its collective breath. In April 2003, the provincial Liberal party, which had campaigned under the leadership of Jean Charest on a platform of improving healthcare, ended nine years of Parti Québécois rule. Charest named Philippe Couillard, a popular neurosurgeon, as his health minister. Couillard, who replaced Charest as party leader in 2013, wasted no time in getting down to business. New legislation was passed. Bill 30 reduced the number of bargaining units in the health and social services sectors and changed the way collective agreements were negotiated. As a result, the 14 labour union locals representing lab technicians and support staff at St. Mary's were merged into four. Bill 31 allowed the hospital to contract out a number of positions, thereby saving money. Bill 25 increased the healthcare budget and abolished the system of regional health boards, replacing them with two new administrative bodies: the Agences de développement de réseaux locaux de services de santé et de services sociaux (CSSS and CLSC), which put the healthcare emphasis on prevention, sanitation, and hygiene; and the Réseaux universitaires intégrés de santé (RUIS), whose role it was to integrate healthcare services on a province-wide basis. St. Mary's was part of the McGill RUIS, and with its official designation as a CHAU still pending, it continued to play an integral role with regard to McGill. More importantly, the new government indicated its appreciation of the fact that St. Mary's had been underfunded by $3.2 million and was carrying a $5 million debt load. Funding was marginally increased, and the hospital's plan to invest $5 million to renovate and expand its dialysis unit was approved.

An outbreak of severe acute respiratory syndrome (SARS) in Toronto that summer motivated St. Mary's to upgrade its isolation rooms and readjust and coordinate its admission policies with other hospitals on the Island of Montreal. Then, in 2004, a *C. difficile* outbreak resulted in some fatalities and raised concerns because some areas of St. Mary's were difficult to control. However, the hospital's handling of the outbreak was considered good compared to that of other hospitals of similar size.

Also that year, the St. Mary's Hospital Foundation reported that since Heward had taken charge, its revenues had increased by 94 percent – due, in large measure, to a $1.5 million grant from the J.W. McConnell Family Foundation for the birthing centre. Renovations to the Family Medicine Centre were completed in 2005. When the building reopened, on September 30, it was christened the Norma and Robert Hayes Pavilion in honour of Richard Renaud's modest and unassuming in-laws. Robert Hayes, who died in 1981, was an inspector in a wire-manufacturing plant; his wife, Norma Morara, the only daughter of an Italian immigrant couple, worked for 25 years as a secretary in a doctor's office and raised four children. The Hayes Pavilion housed the women's clinic, psychiatric outpatient services, and the ophthalmology clinic, which were donated by the Steinberg family. The layout included spaces for children to play and allowed mothers to breast-feed, creating a family-oriented environment.

Residency training at the centre was under the direction of Alan Pavilanis, an associate professor at McGill. Born in France of Lithuanian parents, Pavilanis was educated in Canada and in the United States. He earned a literature degree from Princeton in 1969 and a medical degree from McGill in 1973. He spent eight years in family practice in the Eastern Townships and served as director of the Adolescent and Youth Medicine Service at the Montreal Children's Hospital. In 1991, he obtained a diploma in epidemiology and biostatistics from McGill while teaching family medicine at Université de Montréal.

The opening ceremony of the Hayes Pavilion was significant because it would be the last time a Roman Catholic cleric was on hand to officiate at the opening of a campus building. Reverend David Fitzpatrick, a retired priest in residence at St. Veronica's Parish in Dorval and a Renaud family friend, was asked to pronounce a blessing. By 2005, only one in five St. Mary's patients claimed to be Roman Catholic; one in five was either Muslim or Hindu, and one in five was Jewish. The remaining did not divulge their religion. Because the hospital was now a multidenominational institution, its Roman Catholic chapel was reconfigured to accommodate people of all faiths, and what had been known as "pastoral services" was renamed "spiritual and religious care." While the sanctuary remained intact, a prayer corner containing no religious statues, icons, or images was built in the nave for those who wanted to meditate in a non-Christian atmosphere.

Sarah Prichard left St. Mary's to take up the position of vice president of scientific affairs and research at Baxter Healthcare in Waukegan, Illinois. Richard Renaud replaced her as board chair. On April 26, 2005, the hospital inaugurated its "crown jewel" – the $2.6 million Birthing Centre. It was the fulfillment of Constant Nucci's lifelong dream. Under the direction of Dr. Robert Hemmings, chief of Obstetrics and Gynecology, the fourth-floor facility featured 13 labour and delivery rooms and enlarged private rooms equipped with jacuzzis. It was and is one of the country's largest and most modern. Now, each year, more than 4,500 babies are delivered at St. Mary's. The centre also serves as a training ground for midwives enrolled at Université du Québec à Trois-Rivières. Hemmings, a gynecologist with a degree from Université de Sherbrooke, worked at the Royal Victoria and Lasalle General hospitals before becoming a chief at St. Mary's.

As the hospital continued to evolve, an ambitious plan to rebuild St. Mary's "from the inside out" was advanced. Joshi again raised the question of university-affiliation status for the hospital, and he and Richard Renaud went to Quebec City just before Christmas expecting to obtain approval for the designation. But the ministry, preoccupied with a provincial election that would reduce the Liberal government to a minority in the spring, again deferred. Although Joshi was unable to nail down the commitment, he remained confident that the designation was coming. He left for China to sign a memorandum of goodwill with a hospital in Enshi, Hubei province; this would allow Chinese doctors specializing in ophthalmology and obstetrics to visit St. Mary's. In keeping with the hospital's commitment to innovative care, the foundation mounted a health and wellness initiative. The Chrysalis Forum would bring together women from corporations and the community for informal meetings on health-related issues. In May, the foundation unveiled a new logo, which it intended to use as a marketing tool: a stylized image of a figure embracing a heart.

The $120 million campus development project was approved by the Center Board in November 2007. The major expansion was slated to involve the addition of two floors to the West Wing, enlargement of the Emergency Department, and renovations to the Intensive Care Unit. All wards were to be converted to accommodate only private and semiprivate rooms in order to reduce hospital-acquired infections. An underground parking lot would be constructed and the medical office building at 5300 Côte-des-Neiges would either be demolished or completely overhauled.

In February 2008, the Cancer Care Program, mandated to provide treatment for four major types of cancer, opened in renovated quarters on the third floor. Almost five years after St. Mary's had applied for university-affiliation status, it finally received official designation from the government. This meant that the hospital was no longer a peripheral unit of the university – it was a vital contributor to McGill's research and training programs. "We had always been a McGill teaching hospital," Joshi pointed out. "What has changed is that now, when I sit at the table with my principal partner, McGill, I no longer sit as a poor cousin. With the ministerial designation, St. Mary's remains autonomous, but it is in a better bargaining position, particularly at the graduate and clinical research levels. It goes without saying that patient care remains the hospital's primary focus."

As a result of the hospital's new designation, two new McGill-funded chairs were established. These chairs were funded by the Hospital Foundation, one being in community cancer care and the

FONDATION DE
L'HÔPITAL
ST. MARY

ST. MARY'S
HOSPITAL
FOUNDATION

The Hospital Foundation has its own identity.

other in family and community medicine research. In January 2010, Jeannie Haggerty was named as the hospital's first chair in Family and Community Medicine research; in April, Susan Law became the hospital's first vice president of Academic Affairs. Michael J. Bonnycastle, who replaced Todd McConnell in 2009 as the hospital's sixth physician-in-chief, said that as a result of the designation, St. Mary's was now a "high-tech, high-touch hospital." Bonnycastle, a native Montrealer who had his tonsils removed at St. Mary's when he was seven, still carried a four-digit hospital card that attested to his lifelong affection for the place. A McGill graduate with degrees in biochemistry and medicine, Bonnycastle was an intern at the hospital in the early 1980s and came to St. Mary's from the Montreal General. "St. Mary's has always kept abreast of developments in technology," he remarked, "but it has never been as preoccupied with politics as larger institutions. Here, we are more involved with patient care."

Richard Levin, former dean of McGill's Faculty of Medicine, observed of the role St. Mary's had begun to play in research and family medicine, "It is ironic that we have arrived at the dawn of the era of personalized medicine, and we mean a 'molecular moment' in which genomics will lead to better health for all. But 'personalized medicine' refers equally to the integration between patient and family physician. In this new world, the family doctor will be the patient's personal guide to their genome on a chip. St. Mary's offers a remarkably rich

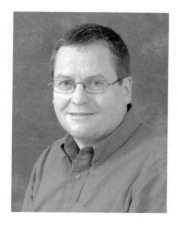

Dr. Michael J. Bonnycastle, the hospital's sixth Physician-in-Chief.

ambiance for research and for [the] capacity to investigate common illnesses and validate therapies, which is critical to the delivery of optimal care in family medicine."

In the spring of 2010, the hospital inaugurated its new dialysis unit. Three times larger than the old unit, it was divided into three areas: a central section with 19 individual treatment stations and 5 semiprivate stations; a peritoneal dialysis clinic; and a renal protection clinic.

CHAPTER THIRTEEN

It's one hell of a success story. The only tools we had to work with at St. Mary's in a highly political atmosphere were people. In a low-level political sense, we were damn good. We have always been ready to bend administrative rules to accommodate our patients, and we succeeded.
~ Larry English

There is something about St. Mary's.

If the hospital didn't exist, someone would have to invent it. In an era of impersonal inner-city hospitals and super-hospitals, St. Mary's remains something of an anomaly: a small, 271-bed institution that has found a niche in a big city. Today it is "catholic" only in the universal sense of the word. It remains a manageable institution where patients experience the personal touch, especially in its obstetrics, oncology, radiology, and family medicine departments. A classic urban hospital, St. Mary's has some 250 physicians on staff and 2,000 employees (nurses and licensed practical nurses, other healthcare professionals and support staff). Every year there are more than 11,000 admissions and 129,000 outpatient visits. The workforce is stable. Like other hospitals, St. Mary's has had to deal with a shortage of nurses; many of those have refused to work overtime.

A certain positive disorder reigns at St. Mary's: everything that needs to get done, gets done, but not in the lineal way one might expect. Patient satisfaction remains high; complaints are few and relatively minor – fewer than 198 a year. With regard to patient satisfaction, Quebec's health minister has put St. Mary's at the top of the list. In March 2007, the French-language magazine *L'actualité* rated St. Mary's as one of the three best hospitals on the Island of Montreal. Similarly, a 2008 *La Presse* survey of the province's birthing centres

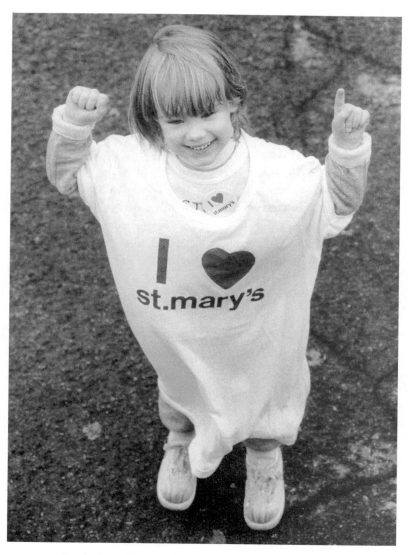

For the love of St. Mary's, four-year-old Melanie Kusicvich demonstrates her enthusiasm. (Photo: Tedd Church)

awarded St. Mary's its highest ranking: five stars. A Quebec government province-wide report card in 2010 graded St. Mary's as the
most efficient and the most underfunded hospital in the province, and
in 2013, the Canadian Institute for Health Information, which monitors health system performance across the country, rated it as one of
the most performant hospitals in Montreal. Accreditation Canada
awarded it an almost perfect score of 95 percent.

If St. Mary's is an exemplary hospital, it didn't happen by accident.
Sometimes referred to as "a mix of good old fighting Irishmen, a fraternity of loyal Loyola College graduates, and dedicated people from
all over the world," it was built on an inspired foundation. Its founders,
Mother Morrissey and Donald Hingston, saw medicine as a mission
and a ministry and not as a business. Sister St. Simon – and legions of
other nuns, nurses, and unpaid volunteers – provided tender care, and
Sister Melanie and Sister Mary Felicitas increased the level of patient
confidence. David Kahn put the hospital on the map after the Second
World War, and John Howlett and Guy Joron forged its links with
McGill University. Richard Moralejo guided the hospital through years
of hectic growth, Constant Nucci upheld the hospital's integrity and
steered clear of expensive scientific projects with short-term appeal,
and Arvind Joshi provided the benefit of his administrative experience
when it was most needed. Then, too, a fraternity of unpaid doctors
who were trained at St. Mary's recognized the importance of teaching
and passed on their talents from generation to generation. In spite
of their professional differences, doctors at St. Mary's are collegial.
They appear to be driven as much by their institutional allegiance as
they are by the demands of medicine and work hard under pressure
because it is the right thing to do.

"As medicine becomes more complex and requires sophisticated
facilities, the larger super-hospitals become places where you can only
teach," explains Richard Cruess, former dean of medicine at McGill
and a core member of the Centre for Medical Education. Cruess
continues:

St. Mary's has always been good in its primary care programs. Up until the end of the twentieth century, teaching hospitals were able to serve simultaneously as academic research institutions while functioning as authentic general hospitals. It was therefore possible for students and trainees to learn both primary care and subspecialty medicine on a single site. This is no longer true. The evolution of the academic health centre into a highly specialized institution primarily concerned with complex issues has made it impossible to teach medicine entirely in these institutions, as the patients being treated no longer demonstrate the breadth of human disease, which every physician must study. Therefore, community hospitals as well as community clinics and primary care physician offices are now essential if we are to pass on the necessary expertise to future generations of doctors. St. Mary's Hospital has always been willing and prepared to go the distance.

Harold Zackon points out, "In terms of the number of specialists we have, it's a fraction of what there are at the bigger hospitals. But to say we are a poor cousin is an exaggeration. The perception is you will get better care at St. Mary's than you do at other hospitals five times the size. It has always astonished me how a hospital with such limited resources has been able to compete."

Let's let a patient have his say as well. Until his death in 2006, Patrick Letang was closely associated with the hospital, first as a janitor, then as a patient. Born at St. Mary's in 1959, he worked there until he became a radio broadcaster. Diagnosed with colorectal cancer, he chose to go to St. Mary's for treatment. Letang attended the St. Mary's Ball in 2006 to help raise money for the new oncology centre. His decision to be treated at St. Mary's, he said, "was a no-brainer. The hospital has never cowered, in spite of the burdens or the challenges it has faced over the years. In a great many ways, it has set the standard for improved medical treatment in all corners. When I think of St. Mary's,

I think of a sign that was displayed in the officer's club in the television series *M.A.S.H.* 'BEST CARE ANYWHERE.' To me, in spite of its limitations, St. Mary's, like the *M.A.S.H.* unit, manages to offer the best care anywhere."

This in spite of constant cost-cutting and uncertain government funding. Quebec government directives issued in 2010 required the hospital to reduce its administrative costs by 10 percent and cut spending on education and public relations by 25 percent. However, in spite of these new financial constraints, at the time of writing, St. Mary's was running a manageable deficit of $5 million and dealing with what McGill's dean of medicine described as "the bitter realities of cash flow." Everything in a health district runs under a single administration, which works well in theory but not always in practice. "St. Mary's comes from a specific community and has a specific role. It is an important place for McGill, but historically, governments are very strategic, and as far as government is concerned, St. Mary's is an outlier, a teaching hospital run by family doctors," says David Eidelman, McGill's current dean of medicine. "Ideally, we would like to see St. Mary's become the headquarters for family medicine, just as the Department of Medicine has its headquarters at the Royal Vic and the oncology department is headquartered at the General." There are concerns, however, that down the road the government could have other ideas and give the hospital another classification within the health district. "If that happens, it certainly would no longer have its own board," says Eidelman. "That would be a disaster, because St. Mary's would no longer be able to chart its own destiny. We are not terribly worried, but we have to be vigilant. St. Mary's has a number of models of care that are superior to a number of other hospitals. It is extremely efficient."

Arvind Joshi prepared a succession strategy aimed at hiring people to usher St. Mary's into a new era, but there have been relatively few changes or additions to the administrative staff in the past two decades. In 2002, Élisabeth Dampolias became coordinator of Human Resources and Patient Information Services; six years later, she was promoted to vice president of Human Resources. Donna Tataryn replaced John Sutton as Surgeon-in-Chief in 2012. Bruce Brown left as vice president of Professional Services in July 2012. He was succeeded by Lucie Opatrny, a Canadian doctor with a master's degree in health-care management from Harvard, the same as Dr. Brown. Opatrny – who is also a specialist in medical problems related to pregnancy and was director of the medical clinic at the International Civil Aviation Organization for five years – had come to St. Mary's from the Royal Victoria Hospital to co-ordinate medical quality. "Among its competitors, St. Mary's is doing better in patient satisfaction and cost efficiency," she says. "Clinically, we provide excellent care, but the immediate challenge is to implement a transparency in our clinical benchmarks so we can have a clear vision and see what needs to be improved."

Early in 2013, Arvind Joshi asked the board not to renew his mandate as chief executive officer. After four four-year terms, he wished to step down with his reputation and integrity intact. "We have taken a competent and a caring hospital, given it stability, and truly positioned it extremely well for the future," he says of his legacy. "Quebec is strong in biotechnology, and it will need strong CHUs and institutes to attract the best technicians, the best academics in the world to maintain its reputation – the people, who, for example, are going to do the first brain transplants. The super-hospitals, in their final format, will have to focus more on tertiary and quaternary care, and less on primary and secondary care. That means there will be a downloading of primary and secondary care patients to St. Mary's. I have no doubt about that. The bad news is that the government doesn't have additional money to give us, and our concern is that the gap is getting bigger."

Dr. Samuel Benaroya, McGill's associate dean of Inter-hospital Affairs and a member of the St. Mary's board, is confident that while St. Mary's "has to act within the financial constraints and the political climate that exists in Quebec," it remains an integral part of McGill's teaching network. A strategic planning exercise has resulted in the establishment of four pillars for it to build upon. "One of our strengths is that we are not a specialty hospital, and, first, we must reinforce our role as a leader in family medicine," says Benaroya. "Second, we take pride in dealing with a multiethnic clientele; we are a beacon for other hospitals in Quebec in that area. Third, we are not alone in the world, so there is a need for participation and for partnership with neighbouring institutions; and, finally, we have to enhance the academic mission of the hospital. The designation of St. Mary's is quite specific. It is a community hospital with academic leanings with important responsibilities in terms of research and teaching."

As St. Mary's prepares to welcome a new generation of leaders, it is hard to find one single word or phrase that will adequately sum up its spirit. Those who have been patients at St. Mary's, those who work there, and those who have been entrusted with running it understand the miracle of a place that every day delivers more than anyone, including its founders, could ever have imagined.

POSTCRIPT

On August 28, 2014, the Board of Directors of St. Mary's Hospital Center announced the appointment of Ralph Dadoun as Director General and CEO.

Ralph Dadoun began his career as a researcher at the Montreal Neurological Institute. A member of St. Mary's staff since 1987, he was Administrative Director of Diagnostic and Therapeutic Services and subsequently Vice-President of Corporate and Support Services, before acting as Interim Director General & CEO since July 2013. A highly respected manager, he has contributed to St. Mary's becoming an important member of the healthcare network.

INDEX

Letang, Patrick xiv, 209-210
Lethal Practice 144
Lévesque, René 142, 151
Levin, Richard 204-205
Liepina, Gerda 80
Lincoln, Larry 183
Love and Success and Other Essays 73
Loyola College 16, 40, 55, 70, 79, 148, 208
Lund, Marie 134
Luhovy, Ihor 127, 156-57
Lynch-Staunton, Hulda 102

MacDonald, Donald 89
MacIntyre, James 45
Macklem, Janet 161
Madore, Pat 109
Maguire, Sister Grace 134
Mahoney, Jean 134, 149
Mance, Jeanne *see* Jeanne Mance
Markham-Stouffville Hospital 185, 190
Marriott Corporation 173
Martel, Marjolaine 140
Martin, Paul Jr. 184
Martin, Paul Sr. 77-78, 86-87
Mary Elaine, Sister *see* Jacobs
Mary Felicitas, Sister *see* Wekel, Sister Mary Felicitas
Mary Lenore, Mother 113
Mason, John Leo Delany 14, 24, 29, 44, 74
Matsumoto, George 81
Maxwell, Edward 22
Mayo Clinic 19-20, 44, 89
McAuley, A.G. "Bert" 45
McConnell Family Foundation 201
McConnell, Todd 188-189, 191-192, 204
McCormack, Helene 149, 168, 192
McCormick, Sister Sharon 134
McCowan, Bridget 23
McCracken, Peter 148-49, 172, 189
McCusker, Jane 177

McDonagh, Father Wilfrid Emmett 33
McDougald, Father 29, 30
McDougald, Wilfrid Laurier 23
McGill Academic Health Sciences Centre 184-85
McGill University; Attitudes of 11; Chairs at, 204; Relationship with St. Mary's 62, 65-67, 69, 83-84, 117, 123, 127-128, 131-132, 137-138, 145-146, 160, 177, 193, 203
McGill University: For the Advancement of Learning 65-66
McGovern, Joseph James "Mac" 14, 44, 49, 54, 64
McGovern, John 54
McGregor, Maurice 120, 122-23
McIndoe, Archibald 47
McKee-Farrar prosthesis 127
McKenna, Leo 40-41
McKenna, Mother Margaret 33-34, 40
McKinley, Catherine 60
McLean, Jessie 72
McLetchie, Norman 91, 157
McShane, Father Gerald 20, 21, 36, 38, 48
Medicare 110, 113-114, 115-116, 119-120, 125, 126, 128-129, 130-131, 154, 163
Melanie, Sister *see* Coligan, Sister Melanie
Mellen, George 88
Menetrez, J. H. 81
Mercier, Jules 114
Mercy, Sister 71
Meredith, Sir Vincent 44
Metric system 127
Meyer, Paul 102, 107
Michaels, George 181
Michener, Roland, Governor General 130
Mohs, Frederic 103
Montreal City and District Savings Bank 1, 12, 16, 63

223

223

index entries